A PATH FORWARD

ECHOES OF A SECOND CHANCE

DAVID MEDANSKY

A Path Forward
Echoes of a Second Chance
Second Edition

Published by:
Executive Books | Tremendous Life Books
P.O. Box 267, Boiling Springs, PA 17007
717-701-8159 | 800-233-2665
www.TremendousLeadership.com

Medical Disclaimer
This book is intended for informational, educational, and inspirational purposes only. It is not intended to diagnose, treat, cure, or prevent any disease, and it is not a substitute for the medical advice of a licensed physician or other qualified healthcare professional. The author is not a licensed medical doctor, registered dietitian, or healthcare practitioner.

Before beginning any new dietary plan, intermittent fasting protocol, exercise program, or other lifestyle change described or implied in this book, readers should consult with their physician or qualified healthcare provider — particularly if they are pregnant or nursing, have a history of an eating disorder, are managing diabetes, heart disease, kidney disease, or any other chronic condition, are taking prescription medications, or are under the age of eighteen.

The dietary practices and weight outcomes described in this book reflect one person's experience. Individual results vary, and no specific outcome is promised, implied, or guaranteed. Readers should not discontinue, alter, or delay any medical treatment or prescribed medication based on information in this book.

Every effort has been made to ensure the accuracy and integrity of the information presented. The author and publisher disclaim any liability for errors, omissions, or any adverse effects, loss, or risk, personal or otherwise, that may result from the use or application of the contents of this book.

Paperback ISBN: 978-1-961202-92-4
eBook ISBN: 978-1-961202-93-1

Editor: Lori Karpman

Printed in the United States of America

MOTIVATE AND INSPIRE OTHERS!

Share this Book

This Book is being given to:

____

Because I care about you and your health,

From:

____

This book is destined to impact countless lives.

For you, the reader, may these pages remind you that no matter where you stand, there is always a path forward.

To those who dare to face their truth and seek renewal. May this story be a lantern on your journey and remind you that healing is always possible.

What Others Are Saying

"Medansky cuts through the myths and lies of the food, weight-loss, and health industries. This book gives you the truth and the courage to act on it."
—Dr. David Friedman, Best-selling, award-winning author of *Food Sanity* and *Funny Bones*

"In *A Path Forward*, David Medansky has combined captivating storytelling, practical advice, and an empowering style that will affirm your commitment to improving your health and reprogram your subconscious mind to make it easier to consistently make healthy choices. A must-read for anyone ready to create lasting change and a better future."
—Hal Elrod, best-selling author of 12 books, including *The Miracle Morning (Updated and Expanded Edition)*

"David Medansky has created more than a book, he's created a call to action. Just as leadership begins with leading ourselves well, true health begins with the daily choices we make. David's wisdom, woven into a powerful story, equips readers to break free from confusion, excuses, and failed attempts, and instead embrace clarity, confidence, and commitment. This book is both inspirational and practical, giving leaders and everyday people alike the tools to live with energy, purpose, and tremendous impact."
—Dr. Tracey C. Jones, President of Tremendous Leadership & Best-Selling Author

"*A Path Forward* is an engaging and powerful parable for our modern age of sedentary and busy (overachieving) lifestyles and convenience foods. Readers will find an engaging story with a weighty (pun intended) and important life-enhancing lessons. This is a must-read for individuals seeking to understand the keys to true health and reclaim ownership of their well-being and prolong their lives."
—Dr. Randall S. Hansen, Advocate, Educator, and Thought-Leader Helping the *World HEAL! Author of Triumph Over Trauma, HEAL!, Heal Yourself,* and *Live Your Best Life*

"David Medansky offers an achievable, realistic, and simple approach for healthy and permanent weight loss that anyone can do."

—Jack Canfield, *New York Times* best-selling co-author of *Chicken Soup for the Soul*®

"David Medansky's *A Path Forward* is like the 8-Minute Abs of healthy living, simple, efficient, and incredibly effective. He strips away the confusion and brings health back to basics with a plan that's sustainable for real people living real lives. This book reminds us that small, consistent steps lead to big, lasting change. Inspiring, practical, and full of heart, it's a must-read for anyone ready to reset their health and energy."
—Jaime Brenkus, National Fitness Hall of Fame Trainer & Creator of the Million selling 8-Minute Abs

"*A Path Forward* is a roadmap for personal transformation that every leader should read. It proves that lasting success begins with health. David Medansky has created a guide that empowers readers to rise above challenges and design a healthier, more purposeful life. This book reminds us that true leadership starts with leading ourselves well. A Path Forward is both inspiring and actionable."
—Linda Fisk, Chairwoman, LeadHERship Global

"David's book really takes stories to the next level! I learned so much with the parables that he put together about health, and each chapter gives you education on how to grow your health and be more cognizant of your health.

A must-read for anyone that's looking to be healthier, feel better, and really change their life!
—Steve Ramona, Podcast Host and Business Connector

"Jim Rohn taught that success is something you attract by the person you become. In *A Path Forward,* David Medansky takes that truth and applies it brilliantly to health. He reminds us that our bodies, like our businesses and relationships, respond to daily discipline, purpose, and consistency. This isn't just a book about losing weight—it's about creating a life of clarity, energy, and fulfillment. *A Path Forward* is a guide for anyone who wants to live with intention and build success from the inside out."
—Kyle Wilson, Founder, Jim Rohn International

"I first met David Medansky at an event in Colorado, where his generosity and heart of service immediately stood out. Having been retired as an accomplished attorney, David was ready to give back—offering his time and wisdom to help others. Within a day of meeting me, he shared legal insight that my own attorney hadn't provided—guidance that helped me close a case in my favor, and revealed the kind of man he truly is: kind, thoughtful, and deeply committed to helping others succeed. That same generosity and integrity flows through his writing. In A Path Forward, David draws upon decades of study, research, and life experience to help readers understand how their relationship with food affects not only their physical health, but also their emotional and spiritual well-being. His words go far beyond the surface of diet and discipline—they invite us to rediscover self-worth, reconnect with our bodies, and heal from the inside out. David's journey from attorney to author is a testament to a man who continues to live a life of purpose—transforming his knowledge and compassion into meaningful contributions that change lives. This book is a gift, born of his desire to serve and to see others overcome health challenges rooted in misunderstanding and disconnection. I highly recommend everything David Medansky creates. His work, like his heart, is filled with generosity, authenticity, and the sincere hope that we each find our own path forward."

—Dr. Tammy De Mirza, The Breakthrough Alchemist®

Table of Contents

Chapter One

The Collapse

Michael stood in his corner office overlooking downtown Chicago. The skyline gleamed in the late afternoon sun. His reflection in the tinted glass window portrayed him as a man looking twenty years older than his age. Deep lines around his eyes, a permanent furrow in his brow, shoulders hunched under the weight of invisible burdens.

The office was pristine. Chrome, leather, glass, an aesthetic that looked good in magazines but felt cold and lifeless at the end of another fourteen-hour day.

Stacks of documents littered his desk, along with half-finished cups of stale coffee. He hadn't eaten lunch, unless you counted the candy bar he'd wolfed down between calls. His assistant, Jamie, had knocked on his door twice to remind him about his daughter's piano recital. Each time, he'd waved her away saying, "*Five more minutes. Just five more.*"

Michael had built Caldwell & Associates from a two-person consulting gig into a powerhouse investment banking firm. The money was *great,* more than he ever imagined possible. Michael was living the dream or so he thought. Now, gazing out the window, he wondered if that dream had become a nightmare.

Reflecting back, he recalled the unforgiving, sad, disappointing look in Sarah's eyes as he slipped into bed at midnight, too tired to speak. In college, he'd tell her his dreams, his fears, their plans for their life. Somewhere along the line, the talking turned to texting. Then to sticky notes on the fridge, *Dinner in the oven. Love you.* That last one felt like muscle memory more than meaning, and he hated himself for that.

If he had listened to Sarah, maybe he would have slowed down, skipped that last round of expansions, the high-stakes acquisitions, the plane trips to far-flung locations, the endless nights staring at spreadsheets long after the house had gone quiet. But he didn't. He couldn't.

He still heard his former business partner, Mitch Jorgenson, asking him that fateful question during their last major board meeting. "When is enough, enough?"

Michael hadn't even hesitated before responding with a smirk. "Never."

The word echoed in his mind like a curse.

That single moment defined everything that followed. When a Fortune 100 competitor offered an astronomical buyout for their firm, enough to retire ten times over,

Mitch was ready to accept. It was a golden parachute. A ticket to freedom. Mitch saw it clearly. Michael subdued by his own ego did not. Or rather, he refused to.

Instead of cashing out, Michael doubled down. Driven by pride and blinded by ambition, he bought out Mitch's interest and took full control of the company. He told himself it was about legacy, about building something that would outlive him. Deep down he knew it was his narcissism that derailed any early departure from the rat race. He couldn't stomach the idea of someone else running the company he'd built from scratch.

Now, years later, Mitch was living in Costa Rica with his wife, paddle-boarding before breakfast and sending postcards from places Michael had never visited. Financially free. Spiritually light. And Michael? He was still a prisoner of the empire he refused to let go of.

The headaches had started last winter. At first, they were mild, a dull throb behind his eyes after too many hours at the screen. Then they intensified. Migraines. Pulsing pain that made him wince under fluorescent lights. He ignored them. Just stress, he told himself. Nothing a few glasses of scotch couldn't dull. But it wasn't just the headaches anymore. He began having dizzy spells, feeling lightheaded, shortness of breath. His heart would pound, palpitations making him grip the edge of his desk until the racing slowed.

Michael scheduled a doctor's appointment. Then canceled it. Twice. He knew the truth.

Admitting the issues meant admitting weakness. He wasn't ready for that.

Sarah saw what he refused to believe. The unopened bottle of blood pressure pills still sat in the medicine cabinet, a silent accusation. She'd found him asleep at his desk more times than she could count. She begged him to take a break. To delegate. To take a vacation, even just a weekend away.

But Michael refused every time.

He was a compulsive competitor. A man who confused material success with love and happiness. Who thought exotic vacations and luxury cars could make up for missed birthdays and empty dinner seats. He failed to understand that what his family really wanted, and desperately needed; something he never gave them: his presence. His time. His affection.

He had chosen the company over his wife. Over his health. Over his family.

And now, with his heart skipping beats and his mind racing, he finally began to question whether winning had been worth the cost.

Michael finally left his office and drove to the auditorium to attend Emily's recital. Sarah gave a sigh of relief when he sat down in the seat next to her.

"I was wondering if you'd show up in time," she said looking directly into his sullen eyes.

"I'm here, aren't I?" He could hear the sharp tone in his voice as soon as the words left his mouth.

Michael glanced at his cell phone for the third time in five minutes, shifting in the narrow auditorium seat, tugging at his suit collar.

"Michael, put your phone away," Sarah pleaded.

"I know, I know. I just need to answer a few emails."

He had promised his wife he'd put his phone away during Emily's recital. However, emails piled up like restless ghosts in his pocket.

"Enough already. Turn your phone off and pay attention. Emily's part is up next."

"Shush," a voice from the patron behind them said.

On stage, Emily's fingers danced over the piano keys. She was twelve years old with chestnut brown hair tucked behind her ears, and shoulders tense in concentration. As Michael focused on her music, his vision blurred.

Straining to keep his eyes open, he forced a smile when Emily stole a shy glance his way from her piano bench. She always looked for him during her performance to make sure he was there.

Michael's head throbbed, the pressure mounting. He shifted again, rolling his shoulders and loosening his tie. Michael felt the same uneasiness as before. Lightheadedness when he climbed stairs, breathlessness for no reason when sitting at his desk working or walking down the street. He could no longer ignore the sensation that something was seriously wrong.

Sarah had sensed Michael was about to pass out so she squeezed his hand. Her touch said *stay with me.*

Michael made one last effort to compose himself.

The final chord faded. Applause rose around him in warm waves. Yet, Michael's own hands barely moved. He felt nauseated. He froze. The auditorium lights seemed to swirl. He felt unstable, even while sitting as he continued to fidget with his tie.

"Michael?" Sarah whispered, her grip tightening.

Michael opened his mouth to speak. Nothing came out. His throat constricted, as if invisible hands had tightened around his voice. *Why can't I speak?*

The room shifted, tilting, first a sway, then a violent lurch. The applause still roared, but now it sounded far away, like a storm beating against thick walls. His chest heaved, but each breath was shallow, unsatisfying, too thin to sustain him. *Just one more breath. Hold it together. Don't let them see. Don't let her see...*

His vision fractured. Faces blurred into shadows until only Emily's remained, clear, painfully clear, framed in light on the stage. Her eyes wide, her lips shaping his name. Fear radiated from her, and the sharp sting of guilt stabbed at him. *I've failed her. I've failed myself.*

Sweat trickled down his temple. His heart pounded like a war drum, merciless, each beat reverberating in his skull. He tried to fight it, to anchor himself, but his strength slipped through him like water through open hands.

The edges of his sight folded inward. Darkness pressed closer. And then he felt it, something final. Not just his body giving way, rather a threshold. A door inside him, heavy and ancient, slamming shut.

So, this is how it ends, he thought. Yet even in that despair, a thought flickered faintly: perhaps it was how something else begins.

The last thing he saw was Emily's face, blurred by tears he hadn't realized were in his eyes. Then the world went black. Michael slumped in his seat, consciousness severed, as if the old life he had clung to had finally collapsed in on itself.

> "There are no regrets in life, only lessons."
>
> —Jennifer Aniston

Chapter Two

The Porch and the Nail

Michael's eyes fluttered open. He was no longer in the auditorium. *What the heck?* he thought.

He sat in a worn wooden rocking chair on a wide porch stretching into dusk. The wood beneath creaked with each gentle sway. The air smelled of pine and something familiar, coffee and old leather.

Before him stretched a wide yard framed by tall oaks. Crickets sang in the distance. Three dogs lay at his feet. Two were alert, watching him; the third whimpering softly, shifting on its haunches.

An old man sat a few feet away in a matching rocker, boots crossed at the ankle, hat tilted back on his head. His eyes were bright beneath a brim darkened by years of sweat and sun.

Michael looked down at the whimpering dog. Its paw scraped at the boards, yet it did not move.

"Am I dead?" Michael asked.

"No, you're not dead. At least not yet."

"Am I dreaming?" Michael asked.

"Maybe you are, then again, maybe you're not," the old man replied.

"Why's the dog whining?" Michael asked, surprised at how clear his voice sounded here.

The old man tilted his hat back further. "He's sittin' on a nail," he drawled.

"A nail? Well... why doesn't he get off the nail?"

The old man's rocker creaked in time with the evening breeze. "Guess it don't hurt bad enough yet."

Michael frowned. The dog moved again, whimpered louder, then settled right back down.

"That's... ridiculous," Michael said, almost to himself.

"Is it?" The old man's eyes glistened. "Is it ridiculous? Have you ever done that yourself?"

Michael opened his mouth to respond but stopped. Images flooded in; the light-headedness he'd ignored, the headaches dulled with Advil, Tylenol, and Ibuprofen, the soda cans stacked in his BMW's backseat. The late-night fast food bags from drive-thru joints such as McDonald's, Jack-in-the-Box, Wendy's, KFC, and Burger King. The promises he made to himself that tomorrow he'd do better. However, as with everyone else, his tomorrow never came.

He bit his tongue and swallowed his pride.

"Yeah," the old man said, as if reading his mind. "Most folks sit on nails their whole lives. Better the pain they know than the effort it takes to stand up."

The dogs beside the whimperer barked once, as if in agreement.

Indignant and irritated, Michael demanded, "Who the hell are you?"

"Me?" the old man responded.

"Yeah, who are you and where am I?"

"Michael, you're being given a second chance. A new path to follow. I'm one of your guides. You'll only be here for a few more minutes. Where you are is not important."

"I don't understand."

"You have been chosen to journey to various mystical places garnering insight, knowledge, and wisdom for living a healthy life to share with souls on a self-destructive path, like yourself."

"Why me?" asked Michael. "I'm not a healthy person. I'm probably one of the least healthy individuals."

"Why not you? You're a starfish."

"What do you mean I'm a starfish?"

"A man is walking along the beach. He comes upon a young girl tossing starfish back into the ocean. He asks her why. She answers, 'The surf is up, and the tide is going out. If I don't throw them back, they'll die."

'Young lady, there are miles and miles of beach and thousands of starfish. You can't possibly make a difference,' he says.

The girl pauses, then picks up another starfish and throws it back into the surf. 'I made a difference for that one,' she says.

Michael looked confused. "I still don't understand what this has to do with me."

"Michael, you're one of the lucky starfish being saved. You're being thrown back into the water."

Michael, not fully understanding the gravity of his situation, muttered, "If I'm so lucky, what am I doing here?"

Just then, a neighbor, Billy Bob, walked past. He waved to the old man, and asked, "Hey, John, how's it going?"

"Same old, same old," John responded. "You out for your daily stroll Billy Bob?"

"Yes, sir. It's a gorgeous day to be sitting inside wasting away."

"Enjoy your walk."

Michael chimed in, "He can't see me?"

"Only the person who visits you will be able to see and hear you," the old man replied.

The old man leaned forward, and in his hands appeared a small leather-bound, pocket-sized journal. The light brown leather was soft and supple in his hands. On the front cover the title "Keys" was written, with a single key below the title.

The key shimmered with a soft, silvery-blue patina, as though it had been forged from droplets gathered at dawn. Its bow took the shape of a teardrop, smooth and fluid, encircling a small, wave-like crest etched in delicate lines. Along the shaft, faint ripples spiraled downward, catching the light like sunlight dancing across a clear stream. The bit was cut in graceful curves rather than sharp edges, evoking the flow of water around stones. The key seemed cool and refreshing, like the essence of a mountain spring, a reminder that life, like the body, thrives when nourished drop by drop.

Holding it out to Michael, the old man said, "Take it. This is for you. The reason why you're here."

Michael hesitated, then accepted the journal. Opening it, Michael flipped to the first page. It was blank.

"What do I do with this?" Michael asked.

"When you are ready, the words you need will reveal themselves. Close the journal and open it again."

Perplexed, Michael closed the book and opened it.

This time, on the first page, the word "Water" appeared. As Michael watched in fascination and awe, more words revealed themselves in illuminated gold ink.

"What is it?" he asked.

"A lesson, more like a rule. Nature must be obeyed, or you will face serious consequences," the old man said.

"Lesson? Rules? About what?" Michael asked confused.

"Michael, do you want to die?"

Without hesitation Michael responded emphatically, "No!"

"Then listen carefully. Nature must be obeyed. You must understand and respect Nature's laws. Start each morning by drinking pure water. No more of those energy drinks, or flavored sodas. From now on, you avoid drinking all soda, diet soda, fruit juices, and fruit flavored beverages."

Michael let out a short, confused laugh. "Water? That's it?"

"That's it," the old man said, a smile creasing his weathered face. "The first step isn't meant to be hard. It's meant to get you off the nail. Most folks never do the small things because they're too busy wishin' for big ones."

He tapped the side of his chair. "Drink water when you wake up. Every day. Before coffee, before excuses. That journal is your reminder to get off the nail."

Michael looked at the journal again. "There's nothing written in it."

The old man tipped his hat, his eyes kind yet firm, piercing through Michael. "Look, son, you need to start each day with a glass of water."

"Why? Why is water so important?"

"Because your body is 60 to 70 percent water. Most of the time you think you're hungry, you're not. You're thirsty. And water is a natural anti-suppressant."

"Yes, but I drink a lot of liquids throughout the day."

"Liquids and water are not the same thing. I think you know that. Water is life. Without it, the strongest body will weaken, the sharpest mind dulls, and the brightest spirit fades." The old man pointed toward the trees beyond the clearing. "Out there, you'll find two trees standing side by side. One strong, green, and full of life. Its roots sip from a steady stream. The other is cracked and brittle. No matter how much sun it gets, it cannot thrive. Why? No water."

Michael felt the weight of the parable. His own choices flashed before him: the sodas, the lattes, the cans of "energy" drinks that never gave energy at all.

The old man's voice softened. "Son, your body's no different from those trees. With water, you'll thrive. Without it, you'll wither. Don't overcomplicate it. Start here. Drink water."

He continued, "When you're ready, the next door will open. But you my friend, have to get off the nail yourself."

The whimpering dog shifted again. This time, it stood, limped a few steps away, and laid down in the cool grass, quiet at last.

Michael felt the light-headedness return. The porch faded into mist. The journal glowed in his hands with a soft, golden light.

When Michael awoke, he found himself standing in a courtyard near a small, well-maintained, yet unassuming hut. The courtyard smelled of incense. The porch and old man, along with his three dogs, were gone. The journal felt incredibly light in his hand. Michael opened it to the first page. Words in illuminated gold script appeared as if being written in real time.

> “Most folks sit on nails their whole lives.
>
> Better the pain they know than the effort it takes to stand up.”

The First Key and Commitment for Health

Drink Pure Water

Today, I will honor my body by choosing the purest form of nourishment.

I will no longer pretend not to know what I know. I will no longer rationalize, delay, or ignore the first and most essential truth about my health: my body is made of water, and water is what it needs.

From this moment forward, I choose to drink pure water; not soda, not energy drinks, not sugar-laced teas, and not chemically colored beverages pretending to be "hydration." These may stimulate me temporarily, but they rob me in the long run of clarity, of energy, and of vitality. No more. The fog in my mind and the ache in my body are not mystery ailments. They are messages. Gentle warnings that I have ignored for too long. I will listen now.

I accept that water is life. Every cell in my body relies on it to function. Every organ depends on it to cleanse and heal. My brain, my heart, my liver; silent laborers working around the clock that require hydration to perform the miracles I take for granted.

I no longer outsource responsibility for my health to others. Not to doctors or prescription medicine. I own my health. I accept my health as my personal obligation. The first act of that obligation is to drink pure water, daily, deliberately, and with gratitude.

From this day forward, I will no longer ask my body to function on empty. I will no longer give muddled signals through artificial drinks or pretend that hydration doesn't matter. I will rise in the morning and gift my body with what it craves most: clean, life-giving water.

I will carry a water bottle not as a chore, but as a symbol. Proof that I have decided to live a healthy lifestyle.

Water is not just a health choice. It is a signal to my subconscious that I am worthy of care. That I am not too busy, too stressed, or too far gone to begin again. Water is my reset button, and I will press it often.

I acknowledge that fatigue, cravings, headaches, and brain fog are not always signs of something wrong with me. Often, they are signs of something missing. And that something is water. Pure water.

I release the lie that I need flavor to enjoy hydration. I release the belief that drinking water is boring or hard. It is simple. It is sacred. It is how I return to myself.

Every time I choose water, I choose clarity over confusion, energy over exhaustion, healing over harm. Every sip is a quiet revolution, a small vote for the life I say I want.

I am not waiting for a diagnosis to act. I am not waiting for a breakdown to rebuild. I choose prevention over regret. I choose nourishment over neglect. I choose life.

From this day forward, I commit to drink pure water as my first and foundational act of wellness. I will not let another day go by where dehydration dims my light. I will rise, sip, and shine. My body, my brain, and my future deserve nothing less.

Drinking water is the first key for my health success. I will honor Nature's law to stay properly hydrated one sip at a time. This is my choice. This is my commitment.

Within moments after reading the page, the words evaporated. Poof. Gone. Michael stashed the journal in his pants pocket and drifted into a deep slumber.

Chapter Three

The Man Who Refused Sugar

Michael squinted against the bright morning light. The courtyard had changed. Gone were the incense and village huts. In their place stood a stone terrace overlooking rolling vineyards that stretched toward a shimmering blue sea. Olive trees twisted from the earth like ancient sculptures. A cool breeze carried the scent of rosemary, grapes, and saltwater. Michael looked around in amazement. "Where am I now?"

"You are exactly where you need to be." The voice came from behind him.

Michael turned.

An elderly man stood beside a low stone wall. He appeared to be well into his eighties, perhaps older. Yet there was nothing frail about him. His posture was straight. His eyes were clear and alert. His movements carried the quiet confidence of someone decades younger. He wore simple Venetian clothing. Nothing extravagant. Nothing that suggested wealth. The man smiled. "Welcome, Michael."

"Who are you?"

"My name is Luigi Cornaro."

Michael frowned.

"Should I know that name?"

Cornaro laughed softly. "Most people don't." The old man gestured toward a nearby stone bench. "But perhaps they should."

Michael sat. Cornaro joined him. For a moment neither man spoke as the vineyards swayed gently in the distance.

Finally, Cornaro broke the silence. "You and I have more in common than you realize."

Michael scoffed, "I doubt that."

"Do you, now?"

Cornaro's smile widened. "I was born into wealth. Venice offered every pleasure imaginable. Rich food. Endless banquets. Fine wine. Entertainment. Comfort. Excess."

Michael listened.

"By the age of thirty-five, I had nearly destroyed myself." Cornaro's smile disappeared. "My body was failing as my health collapsed. Physicians believed I would die young."

Michael felt his stomach tighten.

Cornaro looked directly into his eyes. "I had become a prisoner of my own appetites. Most people aren't starving. They're drowning in abundance."

The words landed harder than Michael expected.

The old man continued. "I spent years chasing pleasure while sacrificing my health. I felt invincible. What I didn't realize was that while I was enjoying life, I was slowly shortening it."

Michael stared at the vineyards. He had a flashback to the late-night drive-thru meals, the energy drinks and candy bars hidden in desk drawers. The skipped walks. Stress and the excuses.

Cornaro nodded as if he could see every memory.

"Does any of this sound familiar?"

Michael didn't answer. He didn't need to.

"Unlike you," Cornaro continued, "I received a warning early enough to change."

"What happened?"

"I listened."

"To what?" Michael asked.

"To the whispers of my soul."

The answer surprised Michael.

"That's it?"

"Most people wait for a heart attack, stroke, diabetes, or cancer before they wake up."

Cornaro pointed toward the horizon. "Nature whispers long before she screams."

The words hung in the air.

"What did you do?" Michael asked.

Cornaro smiled. "I simplified."

"That's all?"

"It was everything."

The old man leaned forward. "I stopped asking what I could add and started asking what I should remove."

"Remove?"

"Less food. Less excess. Less indulgence."

He pointed toward the vineyards. "More walking. More simplicity. More gratitude."

Michael shook his head.

"That sounds too easy."

"Exactly."

Cornaro laughed. "People do not struggle because health is difficult."

He tapped Michael lightly on the chest. "They struggle because simplicity feels too ordinary."

For several moments neither spoke.

Then Cornaro said, "Let me tell you a story."

Michael sighed. "Another story?"

Cornaro smiled. "The best lessons arrive disguised as stories. This one involves a man named Gandhi."

Michael recognized the name immediately.

Cornaro began, "A mother brought her son to Gandhi. 'Gandhi, please tell my son to stop eating sugar. It's bad for him.' Gandhi replied, 'Come back in two weeks.' The mother was confused. Her son was thrilled. The woman returned two weeks later. Gandhi said to the boy, 'Stop eating sugar. It's bad for you.'

'Why didn't you tell him that the first time?' the mother asked, slightly agitated.

Gandhi replied, 'Because before I told your son to stop eating sugar, I had to stop myself.'"

Cornaro's eyes brightened.

Michael nodded slowly. "Lead by example."

"Exactly." Cornaro pointed at him. "You know what you should be doing."

Michael said nothing.

"You've known for years."

Still nothing.

"The question is not whether you know." Cornaro leaned closer. "The question is whether you're willing to do what you already know."

The breeze shifted. A cluster of grapes hung from a nearby vine. Cornaro plucked one and rolled it between his fingers. "The problem is not sugar."

Michael looked surprised. "What?"

"The problem is excess." Cornaro squeezed the grape. Juice ran down his hand. "For centuries people have found new ways to overconsume."

"Today it's sugar, ultra-processed foods, convenience, and eating without thought." Cornaro tossed the grape into the grass. "Sugar is simply the modern face of an ancient problem." He reached into his pocket and removed a small golden key and held it in his palm. Unlike the first key, this one resembled a twisting grapevine. Delicate leaves wrapped around the shaft. Tiny clusters of grapes formed the bow. Cornaro whispered, "The second key," as he offered it to Michael.

Michael accepted it. The metal felt warm in his hand. "What does it open?"

Cornaro smiled. "The same thing every key opens."

"The next door?"

"No." Cornaro placed his hand on Michael's chest. "Your willingness to change."

The key began glowing. The journal appeared in Michael's hands. As before, the golden key dissolved into streams of light and flowed into the cover.

The vineyards glowed in the afternoon sun. Cornaro stood. "The world will always offer more. More food. More convenience. More excuses." He smiled. "Health begins when you discover that enough is enough."

The words struck Michael like a hammer. *Enough.*

The same question his former partner had asked years earlier. When is enough, enough? For the first time in his life, Michael wondered if he had finally found the answer.

The journal opened by itself. Words appeared across the page.

Rule Two: Refuse Sugar and Ultra-Processed Foods.

Michael's eyes widened.

The words shimmered on the page like liquid gold. For several moments he simply stared. "That's it?" he asked.

Cornaro smiled. "Simple does not mean insignificant."

Michael looked up. "I expected something more complicated."

"Most people do."

Cornaro folded his hands behind his back and slowly walked toward the edge of the terrace. "People spend their lives searching for complicated solutions to problems created by simple choices."

The vineyards stretched toward the horizon. "The truth is that health is rarely lost all at once." Cornaro stopped beside an olive tree. "It is surrendered one meal, one habit, and one compromise at a time."

Michael glanced back at the journal.

Refuse Sugar and Ultra-Processed Foods.

The instruction felt almost too simple.

Cornaro smiled. "Let me tell you another story."

Michael shook his head and laughed. "I should have known."

"Many years ago, there was a village known throughout the region for its health."

"The people worked hard. They grew food. They cooked meals together. They remained active throughout their lives."

Michael listened carefully.

"Then one day a merchant arrived."

Cornaro's expression darkened. "He brought brightly colored packages. Foods that lasted for months. Foods that required little effort. Foods engineered to be irresistible."

Michael pictured grocery store aisles filled with cookies, crackers, candy, chips, breakfast cereals, frozen dinners, protein bars, and energy drinks.

"At first the villagers celebrated. The food was convenient and inexpensive. Better yet, it tasted good."

Cornaro knelt and picked up a handful of soil.

"The merchant promised freedom."

He opened his hand allowing the dirt to slip through his fingers. "But what he really sold was dependence."

Michael watched silently.

"Over time the villagers stopped growing food. They stopped cooking. They forgot what real food looked and tasted like. Grandmothers stopped teaching recipes. Children stopped asking where food came from. The convenience remained. Their vitality disappeared."

Cornaro stood. "The greatest danger was not the food."

"It wasn't?"

"No. The greatest danger was forgetting what nourishment meant."

Michael felt the truth of the statement. How many things had he accepted simply because everyone else accepted them?

Cornaro pointed toward the vineyards. "Nature provides food."

He then pointed toward the distant city. "Factories provide products. They are not the same thing."

Michael stared at the journal.

For the first time, Rule Two felt larger than sugar. It felt like a choice between nature and convenience. Between intention and habit. Between life and drift.

Cornaro smiled. “But there is another mistake people make.”

“What mistake?”

Cornaro smiled. “But excess isn’t the only trap. Many people make the opposite mistake. They believe one healthy habit excuses every unhealthy one.”

Footsteps echoed along the stone path. A tall man appeared wearing running shorts and a windbreaker. His smile was easy. His eyes were bright.

Michael stared.

“Jim Fixx?” The man laughed.

“The father of the running craze who died of a massive heart attack at fifty-two?” Michael asked.

Jim extended his hand.

“That’s me.”

Cornaro nodded toward the newcomer. “Jim learned his lesson too late.”

Jim looked toward the vineyards. “I believed exercise could save me from everything else.”

Michael listened.

“I quit smoking and started running. I lost weight and felt great. People thought I was healthy.”

Jim paused. “So did I.”

The smile disappeared. “Fitness and health are not the same thing.”

Michael thought about his own life. Periods of exercise. Periods of neglect. Always believing he could make up for bad choices later.

Jim nodded. "You cannot outrun a poor diet. You cannot outrun stress. And you certainly cannot outrun self-destruction."

The statement hung in the air.

Jim smiled again. "Let me tell you a story."

Michael sighed, "Another one?"

Jim laughed.

"You're collecting keys. Stories are part of the price."

Cornaro chuckled.

Jim continued. "A famous chef's daughter complained that life was unfair. Every time she solved one problem, another appeared."

Michael nodded. That sounded familiar.

"The chef filled three pots with boiling water. He placed potatoes in the first. Eggs in the second. Coffee beans in the third. When he removed them, everything had changed."

Jim paused. "The potatoes entered strong and came out soft. The eggs entered fragile and came out hard. The coffee transformed the water itself."

Michael smiled. He knew where this was going.

Jim pointed toward him. "So, Michael, which are you?"

Michael looked down. The question felt uncomfortably personal.

Jim continued. "When adversity arrives, do you become weaker? Do you harden? Or do you transform the situation itself?"

The vineyards fell silent. Cornaro stood beside him. Jim stood on the other side.

Michael thought for a moment. *One man who nearly died from excess. One man who believed exercise alone was enough. Both carrying scars from lessons learned too late.*

Cornaro placed a hand on Michael's shoulder. "Health is not built by dramatic changes." Cornaro smiled. "Choose simplicity."

Jim nodded. "Choose consistency."

Michael looked down at the journal. For the first time, neither sounded complicated.

Cornaro stepped back. "Knowledge changes nothing."

Jim nodded. "Commitment changes everything."

Michael took a deep breath. The pages began glowing. Golden light spread across the paper. New words slowly appeared: *The Second Key and Commitment for Health*

Refuse Refined Sugar and Ultra-Processed Foods. He began to read.

> "Avoid refined sugar, ultra processed,
> and manufactured food.
> These are food imposters."

The Second Key and Commitment for Health

Refuse Refined Sugar

Today, I reclaim my power by refusing the poison that pretends to be nourishment.

I no longer will be fooled by sweet lies. Sugar is not my reward, my comfort, or friend. It is a thief stealing energy, hijacking taste buds, clouding my mind, seducing my will. No more.

From now on, I refuse refined sugar, not out of deprivation, but as an act of freedom. Avoiding sugar is not punishment; it is power. I do not say "no" because I have to, I say "no" because I can.

I have learned the truth: sugar is addictive. Food products are engineered to override instincts and enslave biology. I am no longer a lab rat or a victim. I will not hand over my health for five seconds of false satisfaction. My cravings are cues, and I can rewrite them.

I no longer will live at the mercy of ingredients I cannot pronounce. I will not be manipulated by packaging or nostalgic jingles. I will not justify the daily indulgences that sabotage my strength. I refuse to feed disease with my own hand.

Each time I say "no" to sugar, I say "yes" to clarity, stability, and lasting energy. My blood sugar will no longer ride a rollercoaster of spikes and crashes. My emotions won't be held hostage by cookies, cakes, and convenience.

I accept that my taste buds may protest. Temptation will knock. My answer is my resolve. As I choose differently, my palate will change, my body will heal, my mind will clear, and my spirit will strengthen.

No longer will I wait for a diagnosis to quit. I do not need a doctor's prescription. Treatment is not the same as a cure. I know the truth; sugar contributes to inflammation, weight gain, mood swings, insulin resistance, and chronic disease. I am not too far gone, and it is not too late. I will begin now.

The discomfort of discipline is far less than the pain of regret. I will not dwell on what I did not know. I do now. And because I do, I will do better. This is not about perfection. It is about progress, a future I almost gave away.

From now on, I commit to avoid refined sugar and manufactured foods. I will not dress up poison and call it a treat. I will not bargain with my body, trading long-term wellness for short-term rushes. I choose nourishment, clarity, and freedom.

The second key for achieving excellent health is to obey Nature's law to avoid "fake foods." And I will honor it one choice at a time.

Chapter Four

The Garden

Michael's mind drifted again.

When he opened his eyes, he was standing at the edge of a vast garden just as dawn broke over the hills. Dew clung to rows of deep green leaves. Somewhere nearby, water trickled through a hand-dug channel.

A man in a straw hat bent over a patch of cabbage, hands steady, his movements deliberate. His denim shirt was faded, gloves stained dark from soil. When he looked up, his eyes were clear and kind, calm like still water, amused like someone who had seen this moment coming.

"You look lost," the man said, his voice raspy yet softened by years of gentleness.

Michael looked down at his shoes, now dusted with earth. "Maybe I am."

The man smiled and waved him over. "Then you're exactly where you need to be. Lost folks tend to find what matters here."

Michael stepped between rows, careful not to crush the young sprouts. The man plucked a sun-warmed ripe tomato from the vine and handed it to him.

"Taste," he said simply.

Michael hesitated, then took a bite. Juice exploded across his tongue. Sweet, tart, rich. Nothing like the pale slices he shoved aside on takeout burgers.

"I forgot tomatoes could taste like that," Michael said, almost ashamed.

The man wiped his hands and leaned back against a rough wooden bench. "Funny, isn't it? People spend billions trying to replicate what the earth already gives freely. Chemists in white lab coats mixing chemicals to create 'flavors,' factories, creating what Nature already has, and marketing teams trying to sell us something that isn't actually food. Still, nothing beats what grows from unspoiled soil, pure water, and sun."

Michael looked around at the vibrant rows, the fruit trees beyond them swaying gently. "It's... simple."

"Health usually is," the man said.

He returned to weeding, moving slow and steady. "They call it 'whole food' now, like it's something new. Your grandparents just called it 'food'."

Michael winced. Images flashed through his mind: foil-wrapped breakfasts, greasy lunch bags, long lines at drive-thrus. Food that left him stuffed yet never satisfied.

"Yes, except it's convenient," Michael protested half-heartedly, as if hoping for an excuse.

The man stopped, looked up, and repeated the word like it tasted bitter. "Convenient. Poison can be convenient too when you don't know what you're swallowing. Son, you're in denial and I don't mean the river in Egypt."

He stood opposite Michael and offered a rough calloused hand. "Jerome Rodale."

"Rodale? I know that name," Michael said. It took a moment, then he remembered, "Prevention Magazine, Mr. Organic?"

"Guilty," the man replied, smiling beneath his straw hat, "I'm impressed you remember who I am."

"I saw you on 'The Dick Cavett Show' as a kid. You talked about living to a hundred."

"And then I died of a heart attack right there on the set. I was only 72," Rodale said plainly, sitting down on the bench.

Michael nodded uncomfortably. "So... why should I listen to you?"

Rodale chuckled. "A fair question. Here's the honest answer. Even when you know what's good for you, knowing isn't the same as doing. That's an entirely different story."

"What happened? Why the heart attack?"

"My mistake was in thinking food alone was enough. Health is a lifestyle, not just what you eat, but how you live. Your movement. Your rest. Your joy. I had the food part mostly right. I ignored my own stress, sleep, and pace."

"But you're the founder of *Prevention Magazine*," Michael exclaimed.

Rodale shrugged. "Many of us think we're healthy when, in fact, we are not. Jim Fixx focused on exercise, not enough on eating right. I focused on real food, ignoring moving my body. And you, Michael, you ignored both."

Michael folded his arms. "I admit I have unhealthy eating habits. So what? Why bother being healthy at this point in my life?"

Rodale replied, "If you can't do it for yourself, do it for Emily and Sarah."

"I suppose you're right." Michael saw a flash of his wife and daughter's loving faces looking back at him. He instantly felt guilty for the way he was harming himself, and in turn, harming them.

Rodale leaned forward, "Michael, it's not your fault, not entirely. The food's changed since you were a kid. It's not as nutrient dense. It's the corners the food companies cut and the deceptive marketing that makes you think what you're eating is good for you."

Without a word, Rodale extended his hand. Resting in his palm was a different kind of key.

This key was slightly larger than the last, forged from a darker metal, glowing warm like aged bronze. The stem was straight and sturdy, but the bow, its head, a sprouting seed, was carved in relief. Tiny leaf etchings climbed, marked by a faint spiral groove, like the helix of a vine. It didn't shimmer; it radiated deeper with earthbound wisdom.

"This," he said, "is the key to life itself. Not to open a door, but to unlock the truth every living thing already knows."

He gestured toward the rows of vegetables, swaying fruit trees, bees in sunlight. "Growth takes time. It needs care. You can't force a seed to sprout by shouting at it. You can't rush a tree to bear fruit by pulling on its branches. Health is the same. It must be nurtured, season by season, choice by choice, until it becomes so rooted that even storms can't shake it."

He looked Michael in the eye, his smile knowing and kind. "This key is a reminder to plant good things in your life. Water them. Protect them. Trust the process. The harvest will come."

Rodale nodded to the journal tucked in Michael's pocket.

"And, what if I don't want to change?" Michael asked. "I'm comfortable with the way things are."

"Comfortable? Seriously Michael? If you don't change, you won't be comfortable. You'll be dead. Or worse, you'll be spending your wealth on illnesses you could have avoided."

"So, it's either change or die?"

Rodale put it plainly, "A person with good health has a thousand dreams. A person with poor health has only one."

Michael pressed the key to the cover. Just beneath the second key, the bronze key melted into the leather like rain into soil. A moment later, the journal flipped open to a new page and golden letters bloomed:

Rule Three: Eat Real Food. Grown, Not Processed. Not Manufactured.

Rodale put a hand on Michael's shoulder. "Food isn't a formula. It's life, energy, intelligence."

Michael nodded.

Rodale continued, "We've let chemistry replace Nature. Now, Nature is calling us back. Before you go, let me share a story about my friend Alex."

Michael nodded, "I'm listening."

"Alex was a master carpenter. He built homes for others his entire life. He poured his heart into his craft. Every nail, every beam, every plank placed with care and pride.

When Alex retired, his boss asked him to build one last house."

Michael listened, already sensing where the story was headed.

Rodale continued, "Tired, Alex rushed, took shortcuts, used cheap materials, did just enough to get by. When he finished, the boss handed him the keys and said, 'This house is yours, Alex, a retirement gift.'

Alex was ashamed. If he'd known he was building his own home, he'd have done it differently."

Michael felt the lesson.

"Your body," Rodale said, "is the last house you'll ever build. No do-overs. No warranties. No refunds. Every bite, every breath, every choice, you're building it daily.

What kind of house are you building? Because if you wear it out, you've got nowhere else to live."

The garden shimmered, bees buzzed louder, Rodale's figure blurred.

Michael was shaken. "Do I get another chance? Is there hope for me?"

Rodale smiled. "You're starting to understand. Rule Three: Eat what is real. What grows. What your body was meant to use. The closer your food is to Nature, the closer your body gets to healing. With every bite or sip, you're choosing to nourish health or nurture disease. Take care of your body as if it matters, because it does."

As the garden faded, Michael closed his eyes. For the first time in years, he felt a sense of relief and joy.

He stood in silence. What kind of house am I building? he wondered. The question settled deep in his mind. He remembered the rushed meals, unhealthy snacks scarfed between meetings, a body that once was an instrument that now felt like a burden. He thought of Emily, of Sarah, and all the moments he wanted to be present for, strong for, alive for.

His hand moved to his pocket, brushing the journal. As he removed it, the journal unfolded itself to a new page. Golden ink shimmered and then burst onto the page with a new message.

> Eat what is real. What grows. What your body was meant to use.
>
> The closer your food is to Nature, the closer your body gets to healing.

The Third Key and Commitment for Health

Eat Real Food

Today, I will build my body with the raw materials Nature intended.

I will no longer pretend that food isn't fuel. It provides my body with power to function optimally, nourishment to heal, to thrive or it can cause it to weaken and break down.

From this moment forward, I choose to eat real food. Whole food. Food that grows in the ground, swims in the sea, or walks the earth, so long as it is unadulterated and untainted by food companies. I will seek food that is as close to its natural form as possible untouched by factories, free of deceitful labels, and uncorrupted by chemicals I cannot pronounce.

I will not be seduced by convenience disguised as nourishment, nor trade my health for packaging, shelf life, or false promises. Just because something is easy to grab does not make it safe to eat.

I know now that food is not created equal. There is a vast difference between what fills me and what nourishes me, between what satisfies my tongue and what sustains my cells.

I accept that food is not for socializing and entertainment. It is not a reward. It is not a remedy for boredom, loneliness, or stress. It is a sacred exchange between the earth and my body. A relationship I have neglected, and one I now choose to restore.

I will honor that relationship. I will ask: Where did this come from? How was it grown? What was added or removed for it to land on my plate? If it had to be modified to survive on a shelf for months, it was never meant to survive in me.

I will no longer be fooled by shiny wrappers or clever advertising. Real food doesn't shout "heart-healthy" or "low-carb," or "immune support." Real food just *is* pure, simple, powerful. That is enough.

From this day forward, I commit to building my body like a master carpenter builds a home...with care, integrity, and quality materials. I will not cut corners, use cheap ingredients, or slap together my meals and expect them to sustain a vibrant life.

Every bite I take is a building block or a wrecking ball. And I choose to build.

I will not seek perfection, only progress. I understand there will be moments of weakness. I will accept them and not make excuses. Each day offers a fresh opportunity to choose differently. I will not let yesterday's choices define tomorrow.

I will forgive my past ignorance and embrace new wisdom. I thank my body for carrying me when I neglected it. Now, I will feed it as if it matters. . . because it does.

From this day forward, I commit to eat real food. I will nourish myself with what grows, what breathes, what lives. I will feed my health, not my cravings.

My commitment is to obey Nature's third rule for my health, to eat real food. And I will honor it one honest bite at a time.

Chapter Five

The Monk and the Meal

Sleep pulled Michael back under like a slow tide returning to the ocean.

When he opened his eyes, the air was cool and fragrant, scented with cedar and steamed rice. He was seated on a flat stone bench in a quiet courtyard. Bamboo rose tall around him, swaying in a slow, silent rhythm. Across from him sat a monk in a simple saffron robe, head shaved, hands folded in his lap. Steam curled gently from a small bowl set between them.

No words. Just stillness.

Michael shifted, clearing his throat. Nothing. The monk remained perfectly still, his gaze soft and steady. In that silence, Michael sensed something sacred, fullness without words.

At Michael's side was a wooden tray with a bowl of rice, a piece of fruit, a cup of water. Simple. Humble. Alive.

The monk gestured, slow and deliberate, inviting Michael to join him.

Michael picked up the bowl. Its warmth surprised him. A tightness sat in his stomach, not from hunger. Rather it was guilt. He remembered all the times he'd inhaled food behind the steering wheel, barely tasting it; lunches scarfed down while reading emails, dinners devoured in front of the TV or at his home office desk. Always rushing. Rarely present.

As a boy, he remembered family dinners. His mother's lasagna, his father's prayer, siblings arguing over who got seconds. There was laughter. Togetherness.

Now he couldn't remember the last time he sat at the dinner table with Sarah and Emily.

The monk lifted his bowl, bowed his head, and breathed in the steam. His eyes fluttered closed.

Michael did his best to mimic him, though he felt ridiculous.

They ate. The monk moved with intention, lifting each spoonful to his mouth, chewing slowly, almost reverently. Michael attempted to match him, but his jaw moved too fast, and his thoughts raced ahead.

The monk paused, raised a hand, and tapped his chest over his heart.

Michael sighed, slowed down and let the rice linger on his tongue. He noticed the warmth, clarity, and sweetness in each bite. The courtyard quieted. Within that silence, Michael felt something unexpected—gratitude.

For the first time in years, he wasn't consuming food. He was nourishing his body.

When they finished, the monk placed his palms together whispering a prayer.

Michael followed, awkward, yet sincere.

Just then, a woman stepped out from between the bamboo. She walked with easy purpose, her eyes calm with knowledge and warmth. She wore a simple, powder blue dress and sat beside the monk as if she had always belonged.

"Hello, Michael," she said. "I'm Adelle Davis."

Michael blinked, "Wait. THE Adelle Davis? The nutritionist?"

The monk nodded. "She came to remind you that food is more than fuel. It's to nurture your body."

Adelle smiled. "And to your family. To your future. Even the world."

Michael frowned. "Pretty big claim for a bowl of rice."

Adelle chuckled. "Michael, people think eating is a chore. Something to rush through. But, when you rush eating your meals, you rush your life. When you dismiss meals, you dismiss yourself."

Michael contemplated her words for a moment, then replied, "I've always been more of a sprinter than a marathoner, especially with food."

"And how is that sprint working out for you?" she asked.

"Touché. Let's just say the finish line keeps getting wider," Michael deadpanned.

Adelle, laughing softly, revealed a smooth, round stone no bigger than a quarter.

Michael turned the stone in his hand. Carved into its surface, in soft curves, was a single word:

Slow.

Adelle leaned closer. "Every bite is a choice. And every choice creates a ripple."

After a moment, Adelle rose and invited Michael to join her on a walk. They wandered to a small pond. "Throw the stone in, Michael," she said.

He hesitated, then tossed it. Ripples spread outward.

"Now," Adelle said, "stop the ripples with your hand."

Michael crouched, swiped at the water, splashed clumsily. The ripples just kept going. Frustrated, he said, "I can't. It's impossible to stop the ripples. Why would you want me to stop them?"

Adelle smiled and asked, "So, you are unable to stop the ripples?"

"Correct."

"That's the point. Every action, every word, every bite you take creates ripples into your life, your health, your family, your business. You can't stop them."

Michael folded his arms. "Okay. I cause ripples in my life. What does that have to do with my lunch?"

Adelle knelt, touching the pond's surface. "You choose the stone you throw. Is it a stone of health? Compromise? Is it nourishment or disease?"

Michael muttered, "And here I thought it was just rice."

Adelle smiled gently. "The ripples go farther than you imagine. Your eating habits ripple through your body and your family."

Michael looked down uneasy. "What does this mean for me?"

Adelle's voice softened, "A person with excellent health has a thousand dreams. A person with poor health has only one, to be healthy."

Michael smirked faintly, "Yeah, I've heard that quote before."

"Then hear this one: you've sacrificed your health in pursuit of wealth. Now, you're spending your wealth in pursuit of health."

Michael bristled, "Well, before today, I was doing just fine."

"Really? Do Sarah and Emily see you as thriving, or as a burden because of your health?"

He opened his mouth to retort, then closed it. The silence that followed felt heavier than words. For once, Michael refrained from justifying his choices. He listened to the world around him.

The pond shimmered in the light, its surface echoing Michael's ripples. The monk stood quietly beside them, an anchor in still water.

Michael's chest ached. *Have I become a burden to Sarah and Emily?* he wondered.

Adelle reached into a small pouch and drew out another key. Unlike the others, this one wasn't metal. It was carved from wood. Dark, smooth, and shaped like a teardrop. Delicate lines were etched into its surface like tiny ripples, radiating out.

She pressed it into Michael's palm.

"This one," she said softly, "was grown, not forged."

Michael felt its warmth. It didn't sparkle; it pulsed with presence.

"This belongs in your journal," she said.

Michael pressed it to the cover and the wood melted into the leather. The journal unfolded to a new page. Gold words bloomed:

Rule Four: Eat Slowly. Choose Peace Over Pace.

The monk spoke gently, "When you eat slowly, you teach the body it is safe. You turn meals into moments. You remind yourself that life, real life, happens between the bites."

Adelle added, "Fast food creates fast lives. And fast lives burn out. Slow is not lazy. Slow is wise. Slow is sacred."

Michael nodded. "Eat slowly. Taste my food. Guess that beats inhaling burgers and fries in the drive thru." He watched the ripples from the stone fade on the pond.

Now, he understood. Michael clutched the journal tighter, its warmth radiating through his palm. He closed his eyes.

When he opened them, the courtyard was gone.

> Eat Slowly.
>
> Choose Peace Over Pace.

The Fourth Key and Commitment for Health

Eat Slowly and Mindfully

Today, I honor my body by being fully present with the food that nourishes it.

No longer will I rush through meals or treat eating as an afterthought. From this moment forward, I choose to eat mindfully, with gratitude, awareness, and intention. I now understand *how* I eat matters as much as *what* I eat and *when* I eat.

I will not eat in front of a screen or behind the wheel. I will not inhale my food out of habit, stress, or distraction. I will slow down. I will chew with presence. I will taste the food that was grown, prepared, and served for my nourishment.

Each bite is a conversation between my body and my life. When I eat in chaos, I digest chaos. When I eat in stillness, I invite healing.

Mindful eating may feel unfamiliar, slow, or awkward. But anything done with reverence becomes sacred. I am not just building new habits. I am building a new relationship with food.

I will not numb myself with food nor use it to escape emotions I'm afraid to feel. I will sit with my hunger and ask what it truly craves. Sometimes it will be nutrient, water, or rest. I will listen and learn the difference.

No longer will I eat because the clock says it's time or the plate is full. I will eat when I am hungry, not bored, anxious, or guilty.

I release the belief that more food means more satisfaction. I release the idea that fullness equals being fulfilled. I will eat until I am nourished.

I will see meals not as interruptions, rather as sacred pauses. Moments to reconnect with my body, ground my spirit, and give thanks for the miracle of digestion. I bless my food, not just with words, but with presence.

I will not shame myself for the past, nor regret rushed meals. I forgive my old self, and now I choose differently.

Mindful eating is not about rules. It's about respect. It is about remembering food is necessary for my body to thrive. When I slow down, I can hear what I once ignored.

From now on, I commit to eat mindfully. I will savor my meals. I will honor the hands that prepared them, the earth that provided them, and the body that receives them.

My commitment is to obey Nature's fourth rule for my health; to eat slowly and mindfully. I will honor it one conscious bite at a time.

Chapter Six

The Banquet

When Michael opened his eyes, the pond and its gentle ripple had vanished. The forest silence dissolved. Now, he sat alone at the far end of an impossibly long banquet table, a glimmering stretch of opulence fading into the distant horizon.

The table sagged under towers of golden bread, rivers of velvety sauces, pyramids of fruit so ripe they practically glowed. Crystal goblets shimmered with light that came from nowhere.

Michael's stomach growled. Not from hunger. Rather, temptation. His body didn't need food. His eyes did.

Then a calm, piercing voice broke the stillness, clear as a bell ringing in a cathedral.

"A man who feeds his stomach more than it needs, feeds his suffering."

Michael turned. A man in crisp white linen approached. His skin radiated health. Not the polished sheen of vanity, but deep, glowing vitality, like someone in complete harmony with Nature. "And you are?"

"Paul Bragg. And you, my friend, have already had enough."

Michael, confused, retorted, "But… I haven't eaten anything."

"Exactly," Paul said, a knowing grin on his face. "Your eyes are hungry, not your body."

He snapped his fingers. The banquet table vanished. In its place, a sprawling pasture appeared, beneath a cloudless blue sky. A chestnut horse galloped freely across the field, its mane streaming like fire.

"That's Thunder," Paul said, nodding toward the magnificent animal. "A thoroughbred. A champion."

They leaned against a split-rail fence as the horse slowed to a canter, then trotted to a stop, breathing easily. The sunlight danced on his coat like liquid bronze.

Moments later, a man waddled into view, winded just from walking. His belly strained the buttons of his shirt like a dam ready to break. He dropped a feed bucket with a grunt.

Thunder trotted over, nibbled a few bites, then walked away, content.

"This," Paul gestured toward Thunder, "is how a champion eats. Enough to fuel. Not to numb. Enough to thrive. Not to escape."

"Yeah, I get it. Fuel, not feast."

The man puffed his chest and started boasting about

Thunder's supplements, vet care, trainers, even dental work. Michael glanced from the horse to the man's belly. The irony struck like lightning.

Paul turned to the big-bellied man, "You know exactly how to keep your horse in peak condition. So, why not treat yourself the same way?"

The man chuckled, rubbing the back of his neck. "Ah, well. Thunder's an athlete. I'm just... me."

As quickly as they appeared, the horse and the man vanished, leaving only Paul and Michael in the pasture.

"What just happened?" Michael asked.

Paul looked at him, "You're not so different. Not from Thunder's owner. Not from most people."

Michael raised a brow. "What do you mean?"

"Do you own a pet? A dog or a cat?"

"No." Michael replied.

"Pity," Paul replied. "Most people feed their pets better than they feed themselves or their kids. They'll buy grain-free, organic dog food, but scarf down fast food without a second thought. Would you give Coke or Pepsi to a dog?"

"Of course not," Michael scoffed.

"Well then, why do you drink that stuff?" Paul asked, direct.

Michael winced. "I have no comeback."

"You're not a trash can, Michael. Stop treating yourself like one." Paul reached into his pocket and pulled out a worn bridle, its metal buckles shining.

Paul handed it to Michael. "Do you know what this is?"

"A bridle."

"That's right. This one is not for the horse. It's for you."

Michael cocked his head. "For me? Unless you're planning on riding me into the sunset, what do you mean?"

"You need to rein in your urges," Paul said calmly. "Hunger is natural. Overindulgence is learned."

Michael examined the bridle. Tiny words were engraved on the buckle:

Small portions.

Paul waved his hand, and suddenly a wooden table appeared; set with two plates, one large, one small.

"Which plate looks like it has more food?" Paul asked.

Michael pointed to the smaller plate, "That one."

Paul smiled. "That's funny because they both have the exact same amount."

Michael looked closer, squinting as it dawned on him. "You're right."

"Our culture praises abundance because it doesn't understand moderation," Paul said. "It's all perception."

"So, the trick is to use a smaller plate?"

"Exactly. And use a blue plate."

Michael exclaimed, "What? Why?"

"Blue suppresses appetite. There are very few naturally blue foods. Your brain doesn't associate it with hunger. Red and yellow stimulate appetite. That's why nearly every fast-food restaurant uses red and yellow. They want you craving more."

"Bastards," Michael muttered.

Paul laughed. "Subtle, isn't it? But powerful. Change the plate, change the color, change the portion, change the message you send to your brain."

The long banquet table reappeared, but now the abundance was gone. In its place were modest portions, clean, intentional servings. No gluttony, no shame. Just nourishment.

Paul stood by Michael, "When you master your portion, you master your power. A bridle doesn't restrain; it guides. Guide your hunger. Don't let it ride you to the grave."

Michael held the leather bridle in his hands. He looked at Paul and asked, "Is there another key?"

Bragg grinned. "Close your hand around it."

As Michael obeyed, he felt the leather shift within his grasp, coil and twist into a warm, burnished metal key.

Its bow formed a perfect circle, within which was etched a detailed bridle, reins flowing like sunrays. Around the edge, finely engraved, were the words: **Rule Five—Master Your Portion.**

On instinct, Michael opened the journal. He laid the key across the page, and the metal glowed with a deep amber light, spreading warmth. The bridle engraving shimmered; the words **Master Your Portion** rose in luminous script, settling into the paper before the key dissolved away.

"A man who feeds his stomach more than it needs, feeds his suffering."

The Fifth Key and Commitment for Health

Eat Small Portions

Today, I honor my body not through quantity, but through quality.

No more will I confuse indulgence with nourishment. I will not eat for entertainment, escape, or ego. I understand now that my power begins where my portions end.

From now on, I eat small portions, deliberately, mindfully, gratefully. I nourish myself to thrive, not to numb. I eat like a thoroughbred; just enough to sustain strength, not to sacrifice performance.

I release the myth that more is better, the belief that fullness equals fulfillment. I do not need to be stuffed to be satisfied or fed to be whole.

My hunger is not my enemy. It is a signal. I will listen, not react. I trust my body to tell me when it's had enough.

Portion control is not about restriction. It's about respect. Every bite is a message to my body: "I care. I'm paying attention. You matter."

I make intentional choices. I will downsize my plate, slow my pace, and eat with presence. A bridle does not punish a horse, it gives direction. I will guide my own appetite with the same wise caring.

No more will I reward stress with sugar, mask emotion with excess, or trade my future for a few more bites.

From today forward, I will master my portion. I choose quality over quantity. Awareness over autopilot. Power over pressure.

Because mastering my portion means reclaiming my clarity, my energy, my life.

My commitment is to Nature's fifth rule for my health; eat smaller portions. And I will honor it one intentional bite at a time.

Chapter Seven

Sleepless Nights

Michael stood frozen outside the hotel room, gripping his key card like it might shatter in his hand. The hallway buzzed with the low murmur of elevators, the soft hum of the ice machine, and the distant ring of a phone. Yet, everything felt suspended in time, as if he was the only person not moving in a world spinning on fast-forward.

He had just finished delivering a keynote speech. A milestone in his career. The applause still echoed in his ears, hollow and artificial, like a soundtrack piped in through speakers.

A little girl passed with a red balloon on a string bobbing behind her. She giggled, carefree in a world not yet burdened with calendars and deadlines. As she turned the corner, the balloon popped.

A sharp crack tore the silence through the hallway.

Michael flinched, like he was jolted with a bolt of electricity. His heart pounded. Something was wrong and he couldn't explain it.

What is wrong with me? he wondered.

As he stumbled into his room, the door slammed shut behind him with a loud thud. Without turning on the light, Michael collapsed face-down onto the bed, still dressed in his suit. The weight of the day pressed into his spine, every limb aching with exhaustion.

He shut his eyes and begged for sleep. Yet, his mind continued to race, refusing to shut down.

He clenched his jaw. The city glow bled through the curtains. It was late. He needed to rest. He couldn't. He tried again to fall asleep.

Nothing.

Images spun through his mind. The applause, his daughter's unread text, the urgent green notifications on his phone, the hotel ceiling with that blinking red light from the smoke detector.

And then, everything shifted.

Suddenly, he wore sandals instead of dress shoes. He stood in a forest.

Soft moss cushioned his feet. Towering trees arched overhead like a living cathedral. Shafts of golden light cut through the green canopy. The air held the scent of cedar, sage, and lavender. It was quiet. Not just around him, but inside him.

A nearby stream burbled over rocks. A warm breeze brought the soft flutter of leaves. An owl called, oddly, in the daylight.

He turned slowly, absorbing the peace.

From behind a tree, a man stepped into view. He appeared older, dignified, and unmistakably grounded. He wore a weathered gray wool suit and carried a carved wooden staff. His expression was kind yet penetrating.

"Michael," the man said, his voice deep and smooth, like river water over stones. "You're running on fumes."

Michael looked into the man's eyes, "Do I... know you?"

"Halbert Dunn," he said with a slight bow. "I'm called the Father of Wellness."

The name clicked. Michael remembered reading about Dunn decades ago. Dunn believed health was more than the absence of disease.

"Where am I?" Michael asked.

"Somewhere quieter than you've been," Dunn replied. "Come. Walk with me."

They started down a sun-splashed path. Birds chirped overhead. The silence between them, though awkward, was restorative.

"You treat sleep like a luxury item, something to indulge in when there's nothing urgent left," Dunn said.

"Because there's always something urgent," Michael muttered. "If I stop to rest, everything falls apart."

Dunn stopped, locking eyes with Michael. "No,

Michael. If you never stop to relax, *you're* the one who falls apart. Rest is a radical act of self-love in a world that glorifies exhaustion."

As they continued walking, Michael contemplated his words. After a few minutes, they came upon a tiny green seedling.

"See that seedling, pull it out," Dunn instructed.

Michael bent, plucked the seedling with a quick yank. Its roots were shallow.

"Now what?" Michael asked.

"Now replace it in the same spot."

Michael did. Farther along they found a knee-high sapling.

"Now pull that one." Dunn ordered.

It took effort. He rocked it, twisted, and eventually wrenched it loose.

Again, Dunn instructed Michael to replace the young tree.

Michael, despite being confused, continued walking with Dunn. Eventually, they approached a mighty oak so tall it blocked out the sky. Its trunk was as thick as a small car. Roots gnarled around it like petrified snakes.

Dunn gestured toward the tree.

"You're not going to ask me to pull this one up too, are you?"

"No, but remember, habits are like tree roots. They start small, barely visible, but run deep with time. They're much harder to change as they grow."

"So I'm entangled by my own bad habits?"

"Not entangled. Just deeply rooted. The good news is you can choose which roots to nurture. Water the healthy ones, starve those that choke you. Start pruning one cut at a time. Go to bed thirty minutes earlier. Turn off your screens; cell phones, TV, computers,"

"Easier said than done. No pun intended."

Dunn laughed.

Michael thought about what Dunn had said. "Protect my sleep. Funny, I've been protecting my deadlines more than my own life."

"Michael, you cannot buy back lost sleep. However, if you give your body rest, it will repay you with mental clarity, strength, and life."

"Alright, doc. I'll trade my work binges for a longer, healthier life."

A breeze rustled through the trees. The temperature dipped. Michael shivered. "What's happening?"

"A shit storm is coming," Dunn replied, eyes narrowing slightly. "It always does. Illness. Grief. Change."

They stopped at a tree scarred by lightning, blackened trunk, but the roots living.

"This is burnout," Dunn said. "Damaged yet still standing because its roots run deep."

"You don't need more willpower. You need profound sleep," Dunn said.

"I know that!" Michael snapped, feeling his exhaustion and desperation all at the same time.

Ignoring Michael's outburst, Dunn replied, "That's the thing about habits, Michael. They run on autopilot. You don't even have to think. Good or bad, they streamline your day." He smiled. "But do things slowly, with meaning, and it becomes a ritual."

"Like brushing my teeth?"

"Exactly."

Dunn bent and picked up something from the ground, pressing it into Michael's hand.

"From this grows the mightiest oak only if planted, protected, and given time."

The acorn was inscribed with the word, **Sleep.** On the other side were the words, **Rule Six.**

"What, no key?" Michael asked.

Dunn chuckled, shaking his head. "Michael, didn't you ever hear the story of Jack and the Beanstalk? Jack thought he was just trading his cow for a handful of beans. But those beans became the doorway to a completely new life. This acorn is your new beginning."

He continued, "Sleep is the foundation of wellness. Without it, everything else, diet, exercise, even your thoughts, will crumble."

"Tell me about it. My brain feels like mush most mornings," Michael replied.

"That's because your body and mind beg for rest. Think of sleep as your repair shop."

"Yeah, but I've got deadlines, emails, a business to run.

Who has time for repair shops? I can barely get the oil changed in my car."

"And what happens to that car when you keep skipping its maintenance?" Dunn asked.

"It breaks down."

"Exactly. You've been driving yourself on fumes. No pit stops. No repairs."

The breeze slowed. The trees stilled. The trees in the forest seemed to lean closer, listening.

Michael's voice was quiet. "So how do I change it?"

"You don't fix sleep. You value and honor it."

He looked up through the canopy, golden light shimmering through the leaves.

"When the dark comes, don't resist. Surrender."

The forest faded to gold. Leaves shimmered, the air stilled. Michael took a full cleansing breath.

Michael turned to Dunn. "Will I see you again?"

Dunn smiled. "Every time you choose rest over rush, yes."

The forest dissolved. The scent of cedar faded. The moss disappeared beneath his feet.

Michael was back in bed, but something had shifted. He placed the acorn on the nightstand beside his journal, turned off the lamp, and closed his eyes. This time, letting sleep come softly.

The acorn pulsed gently with ancient light, and unseen to Michael, melded into the journal merging with the other keys.

> “You don’t fix sleep.
>
> You value and honor it.”

The Sixth Key and Commitment for Health

Sleep

Today, I will honor sleep and rest as a sacred act of healing, not a weakness to overcome.

No longer will I wear exhaustion like a badge of honor. Fatigue isn't productive. Burnout is no measure of dedication. From now on, I choose to sleep not as reward for finishing my work, but because I am worthy of restoration.

Sleep isn't wasted time. It is repair. It is reset. It is the quiet miracle by which my body heals, brain rewires, spirit finds calm. I'll no longer treat sleep as optional. It is foundational.

I understand now that my sleeplessness is not noble. It's neglect disguised as commitment. I won't chase goals on empty. I'll no longer silence my body's warnings. I will listen. I will respond. I will rest.

From today on, I release the toxic cycle of "just one more thing." I release the myth that I can cheat sleep and avoid consequences. I cannot. The human body is not just an incredible machine, it's a garden. It must be tended, watered, and allowed to rest in the dark so it can bloom in the light.

I'll trade nightly chaos for evening calm. I'll create rituals, not routines; rhythms that signal safety, and welcome rest. I'll dim lights, quiet noise, and protect the hours where sleep takes root.

I know rest is resistance. In a world addicted to urgency, rest is my rebellion. When I sleep, I heal, I become whole.

Sleep is not an afterthought. It is a law of Nature; one I must obey.

I won't reach for caffeine for fake alertness or rely on adrenaline to drag me through my day. I won't force my body to perform without recovery. I'll acknowledge the brilliance of my biology the way my cells regenerate, memory consolidates, hormones balance, as I rest.

From now on, I commit to sleep more. I'll make it a priority, not a luxury. I will guard my rest with environments, rituals, and rhythms that welcome it. Because when I sleep well, I live well. And when I honor sleep, I honor life.

And I will honor it, one sacred night at a time.

Chapter Eight

Rest to Digest

Michael stood on cracked ground under a pale, silver sky. The air was still, as if holding its breath before a storm. The landscape felt ancient; half desert, half forest, with rocks jutting up and gnarled olive trees in silent contemplation.

Ahead, a narrow stone path led to a low, domed structure, a humble hut, made of sun-bleached clay, its arched doorway like the mouth of a cave. Drawn by reverence, not curiosity, Michael stepped forward, sensing something waiting for him inside.

Inside, the air cooled instantly. Shadows flickered on the round walls from a fire in the hearth. Jars of dried herbs lined shelves, and the scent of thyme and rosemary lingered like a prayer.

A man stood at the hearth, stirring a pot of something earthy and warm.

"You must be Michael," the man said, without turning.

Michael did not recognize the voice, deep and patient like still water.

The man turned, and revealed a long face, lined with wisdom. His beard streaked with silver; his eyes held the gravity of centuries.

"Hippocrates," he said simply.

Michael's breath caught. "THE Hippocrates?"

"The same," Hippocrates said with a gentle smile. "Father of Medicine. But I prefer 'student.' Always learning. Always listening to the body."

Michael stepped closer. "Where am I?"

"In a space between knowledge and healing," Hippocrates said. "You've learned about what to eat, how to eat, and even how to sleep. Now, it is time to learn when, and when not, to eat."

He motioned for Michael to sit on a smooth stone bench. Hippocrates ladled broth into two wooden bowls and handed one to Michael.

"I thought this would be about food," Michael said, accepting the bowl.

"It is," Hippocrates replied, sitting beside him. "Just not as you expected. Digestion is more than what goes in. It's also about when to allow your body to process it."

Michael sipped the broth, simple yet deeply satisfying.

"People today eat around the clock," Hippocrates continued. "Snacks between meals. Late-night indulgences. Breakfast before dawn. Grazing as if your stomach has no rhythm."

Michael lowered the bowl. “I thought eating more frequently kept metabolism going.”

Hippocrates chuckled. “A myth, sold by industries that profit from your cravings. The body is designed for periods of nourishment and periods of restoration. Without pause, the system breaks down.”

Standing, Hippocrates crossed the room to a wooden table and lifted a humming key from a small box. Its warm, polished surface glowed with an etched sun rising and setting in eternal motion, and along one edge inscribed: **Intermittent Fasting.** The reverse: **Rule Seven.**

He looked into Michael’s eyes. “Rule Seven: Rest to Digest. Give your body time to cleanse, repair, heal. Eat within a time window. Let your body fast, not as punishment, rather as a gift.”

Michael nodded, though uncertain.

Hippocrates noticed Michael’s hesitance. “Let me put it another way.” He poured broth into a cup and repeatedly poured, swirled, and dumped it into a sink, each time leaving a residue.

“Imagine this sink is your digestive system,” he explained. “Keep adding more meals, snacks, late-night bites. But you never stop to clean out what’s there.”

Michael peered at the dirty sink.

Hippocrates continued, “Eventually it overflows. A stench forms. Decay breeds infection. Soon, you’re not nourishing. You’re overburdening. When you fast, you let the sink, ‘your body,’ drain and clean. You’re not starving. You’re cleaning.”

"You mean, like, it fixes itself just by skipping dinner? Sounds like wishful thinking."

Hippocrates dried his hands, stepped outside, and returned with an olive press. "This press extracts oil. But overuse clogs it. Pulp builds up. If we don't pause and clean it, it slows, then stops."

"Your body is like this press, Michael. Constant food in, no cleaning out, soon, you choke the system meant to nourish you."

"So, my stomach needs a vacation?" The lesson started to make sense.

"Exactly. Clear the buildup, and you'll run smooth again."

Hippocrates scraped out the excess skins, pits, and rinds. He then turned the crank. The stones rolled effortlessly again.

"But what if I get hungry?"

"You will. Hunger is the body knocking, but it's rarely an emergency."

"Tell that to my stomach at midnight," Michael groaned.

"Remember: Fasting isn't starvation. It's the necessary flip side of eating. Healing happens there. Your stomach is exhausted."

"How long do I fast?"

"Start simply. Twelve hours between dinner and breakfast. Eventually, stretch to fourteen, even sixteen. Let your body adapt. Healing happens from both dietary intake and times without food."

The fire flickered. Michael realized he'd always pushed his body too hard, too fast, too often.

"Do you know what the word 'breakfast' means, Michael?" Hippocrates asked.

"To break the fast," Michael said.

"Exactly. Not to start eating, but to end the healing window."

Michael was quiet. "I think... I've been afraid of that space."

"Stillness scares those who find their worth in motion. But healing lives in the silence between meals."

Hippocrates pressed two fingers to Michael's temple. "You do not need more food. You need more rest. Not only for your meal, but for your life."

As the hut faded, the scent of herbs lingered. The key grew warmer in his hand as he returned to himself.

He opened the journal, pressed the sun-engraved key to an open page, and watched as the words **Intermittent Fasting** and **Rule Seven** glowed and then dissolved into the parchment.

He felt a measured, steady pulse of a body finally allowed to rest.

> “Stillness scares those who find their worth in motion. But healing lives in the silence between meals.”

The Seventh Key and Commitment for Health

Rest to Digest

Today, I will honor the rhythm of my body by giving it space to rest, repair, and rejuvenate.

No longer will I treat my digestive system as a garbage disposal or eat as if my body is a machine made for endless consumption. Healing requires pause. Wholeness needs space. Restoration requires rhythm.

From this moment, I choose to rest to digest. I will not feed my body around the clock and call it nourishment. I will allow time between meals for digestion, cleansing, and rejuvenation.

I release the lie that eating frequently makes me healthy, the myth that constant grazing is caring for my body. Instead, I see it for what it is: overload, overindulgence, and gluttony.

Every meal sends a message to my body. But so does every break. When I fast between meals, I let my body do what it is brilliantly designed for; to clean, balance, and repair. That's where healing begins.

I will not fear hunger or fill emptiness just to avoid discomfort. I will listen. I will wait. Stillness is where restoration begins.

I see now that fasting is not starvation. It is structure and wisdom, returning to my natural cadence: eat, then fast. Work, then recover.

From this day forward, I'll give my digestive system the gift of time. I'll fast overnight and let my body adapt. I won't break my fast by the clock, but when my body is ready, the cycle completed.

I'll ignore advertising noise and the pull of late-night cravings. I'll honor the silence between meals, for my body, mind, soul, and life.

When I rest to digest, I make space for wisdom, clarity, balance, and peace.

From now on, I commit to rest to digest. I will nourish with intention and pause with purpose. I trust the rhythms encoded within me. I honor my body's need for balance.

This is my decision. This is my commitment. This is Nature's seventh law for my health. And I will honor it one intentional pause at a time.

Chapter Nine

The River of Stress

Michael had just begun to understand how the body could be strengthened through simple choices such as choosing water over soda, resting instead of pushing past exhaustion, eating real food instead of grabbing what came in boxes or wrappers. Now, another truth pressed. His mind carried battles, invisible but powerful, shaping everything beneath the surface.

Michael stood on a stone embankment overlooking an ancient city unlike anything he had ever seen. Massive walls stretched toward the horizon. Golden towers rose above crowded streets. Merchants shouted from marketplaces. Soldiers marched through enormous gates. The city pulsed with an unbounded energy.

That's when he heard the rushing water. At first, he thought it was rain. Then he realized it was something much larger. A river. A massive river. The water surged past with relentless power, carrying branches, leaves, and debris downstream. Its surface glittered beneath a blazing sun.

Michael stepped closer. The force of the water surprised him. It never stopped. It never rested. It simply pushed everything in its path forward.

"What is this place?" Michael wondered out loud.

"Babylon. Impressive, isn't it?"

Michael turned. A young man stood nearby. Calm, steady, unshaken. Despite the roaring water, he appeared completely at peace.

"Daniel," The young man smiled. "You've heard of me."

"Of course."

Daniel looked back toward the river. "Then you know about the lions."

Michael nodded. "The lion's den."

"You know about the dreams. King Nebuchadnezzar?" Daniel smiled.

"Most people know those stories."

He pointed toward the river. "Very few understand this one."

Michael watched a branch spin through the current. "I thought stress was the problem."

Daniel picked up a leaf and dropped it into the water. Within seconds it disappeared downstream.

"What happened?"

"It drifted away."

Daniel nodded. "Exactly."

The two stood silently watching the river.

Finally, Daniel spoke. "Tell me, Michael. Were you always unhealthy?"

"No."

"Were you always exhausted?"

"No."

"Were you always fifty pounds overweight?"

Michael looked away. "No."

Daniel pointed toward the river. "Then how did you get there?"

Michael opened his mouth. Then stopped. Because he didn't know. Or perhaps he did. One skipped walk, one fast-food meal, an energy drink, a late night, the stressful week.

Daniel smiled.

"You drifted."

The word landed hard.

Michael stared at the water.

Daniel continued. "Most people imagine their biggest problems arrive like storms. They don't. They arrive like currents."

The river roared beside them. Michael watched another branch disappear downstream.

"So, what does this have to do with stress?"

Daniel laughed softly. "Everything."

He pointed toward the river. "Stress is a current."

Michael's brow furrowed, "I thought stress was the problem."

Daniel shook his head, "No."

The current continued rushing past.

"Stress is unavoidable. I lived in Babylon." Daniel smiled. "Trust me. I understand stress."

Michael laughed. "Fair point."

Daniel continued, "When I was taken from my home, my future was uncertain. I lived under powerful kings. I served in a foreign land and faced execution. I was thrown into a den of lions."

Daniel looked directly at him. "If stress alone destroyed people, I would not be standing here."

Michael considered that. "So, what destroys people?"

Daniel pointed toward the water. "Their response to stress, how they react."

The answer surprised him.

Daniel picked up another leaf. "The river carries two currents. One pulls you under. The other teaches you to swim. The river never disappears. The choice is which current you enter. When people are stressed, they stop choosing."

He released the leaf. The river immediately claimed it. The leaf disappeared.

"Some seek comfort."

Another leaf. "Others seek convenience."

Another leaf. "Many seek escape."

Daniel watched another leaf disappear downstream. "Stress has a way of whispering. You've had a hard day. Skip the walk. Order the burger. Have the drink, you deserve it.

Daniel smiled. "Stress is a skilled negotiator. It never asks for everything. Just this one choice. Just this one shortcut. Just this one exception."

Michael felt exposed. Daniel had just described half his life.

The young man smiled kindly. "You see, stress rarely destroys health directly. It pushes people toward choices that do. The king's table was not offered as a trap." Daniel watched the river. "It was offered as a reward. Most compromises are."

The river suddenly appeared wider, stronger, more dangerous. Daniel pointed toward the opposite bank. "Do you know how my story began?"

"The lions' den?"

Daniel laughed. "No, the king's table."

Michael looked confused.

"The food?"

"Yes." Daniel nodded. "Everyone remembers the lions. Few remember lunch."

The statement made Michael smile.

"When I arrived in Babylon, the king offered me the finest food in the kingdom."

"Sounds like a good thing."

"Most people thought so."

Daniel picked up a stone. "The food wasn't the test."

He tossed the stone into the river. "The pressure was."

"What pressure?"

"Pressure to fit in. Pressure to conform. Pressure to become like everyone else."

The ripples spread across the water.

Daniel looked directly at Michael. *"Stress always invites compromise."*

Silence followed. It felt important.

The river rushed past.

Daniel continued. "The easiest thing would have been to eat what everyone else ate. But I chose another direction."

Michael stared at the water.

"So that's the lesson?"

Daniel smiled. "Partly."

He pointed to a branch spinning helplessly in the current. "Do you know why it drifts?"

"Because the river is stronger."

Daniel shook his head. "No. Because it surrendered."

The words hit Michael harder than anything else he had heard. He thought about the years. The choices. The excuses and justification.

Daniel stepped beside him.

"The current will always exist. Stress will always exist. Pressure will always exist."

The river thundered.

"But direction is still a choice."

Michael looked across the water. For the first time he understood. Stress wasn't the enemy. Stress wasn't drowning him. The river had never chosen for him.

Daniel placed a hand on his shoulder. "Stress reveals the direction you've chosen."

The river faded into mist. Daniel's figure blurred, his final words echoing.

Michael watched the current one last time. For years he had blamed stress. The river had never forced him downstream. He had stepped into it willingly.

Michael realized that eating fast foods or comfort foods when distressed was like stepping into the raging current, every bite pulling him further from clarity and strength. He decided, *In the moment of stress, I will never reach for comfort food, Food is not my escape. It is not the solution.*

> "One current, Distress, erodes and drowns you. The other, Eustress, pushes you forward, making you stronger.
>
> The river never disappears, but you can choose which current to enter."

Chapter Ten

Think Positive

Michael's eyes opened to the early light of a city not quite his own, yet strangely familiar. The skyline shimmered with morning mist, the rumble of taxis and buses echoed across streets. He stood at the edge of a Manhattan park, but it was clearly another time; perhaps the 1940s. Life moved slower. Everything carried the smell of ink, wool, and steam.

All around him were signs. Not billboards, but hand-painted words on brick buildings, subway pillars, even lampposts. Instead of selling soap or cigarettes, they were affirmations:

"You are capable."

"Start with hope."

"Your faith is stronger than fear."

Michael wandered the quiet streets, the city waking around him. Church bells rang in the distance.

A man in a dark overcoat approached, fedora perfectly in place, eyes warm, and his voice even warmer. “You’re not lost, Michael. You’re just looking in the wrong place.”

“Do I know you?” Michael asked.

“Norman Vincent Peale,” the man said, extending his hand. “I’m a minister, but I’m not here to preach.”

Michael shook his hand, surprised by the confident grip. “What do you mean?” he asked.

Peale replied. “There was a woman who dropped her keys while walking in the dark. Rather than searching in the dark where she lost them, she searched beneath the streetlight where it was easy to see.

Several neighbors, including myself and other folks passing by, offered to help. After a few minutes none of us could find the keys. Finally, I asked, ‘Lady, where exactly did you drop your keys? We’ve covered every inch around here!’

The woman pointed to an area in the darkness about five feet away.

‘Then why in the world are we looking over here?’ I asked.

The lady replied, ‘Because the light is so much better here.’

Michael interrupted, “Hey, Mr. Peale, I’m not ready to go toward the light. What are you saying?”

Peale continued, “People look for quick fixes, but true health isn’t about doing more. It’s about doing what matters, consistently. Americans spend trillions on health yet remain unwell. The system treats symptoms, not the root causes. Treatment is different than curing."

"I'm beginning to grasp your lesson," Michael replied, his expression shifting as the man's words began to sink in.

"Come, let's walk for a spell," Peale said. They wandered toward Marble Collegiate Church, its Gothic spire rising above Fifth Avenue.

"This city runs on faith. Faith in buildings, in bridges. But what good is faith in the outside world if you lose faith on the inside?"

They entered the church, sunlight pouring through stained glass windows, the sanctuary silent, except for the city's hum in the background.

"Positive thinking isn't pretending problems don't exist," Peale said. "It's not letting them control your mind."

They strolled into a courtyard filled with flowers, benches, and handwritten quotes tucked into stone cracks.

"Let's sit for a spell," Peale said as he sat down on a bench.

"Let me tell you a story about two frogs," Peale began. "Several frogs were hopping through the forest when two of them fell into a deep pit. The other frogs stood around the pit looking down at their friends. Seeing how deep the pit was, they realized they could not help them. There was no hope.

Not wanting to die, the two frogs ignored the others and began jumping as high as they could to get out of the dark and dreary pit.

The frogs at the top of the pit continued to tell the frogs in the pit to give up, as there was no way they could jump out.

After jumping as high as they could over and over, one of the frogs listened to the others and gave up. He accepted the fate of his death and settled into the mud at the bottom of the pit.

The other frog, however, continued with all his might. The crowd of frogs yelled down the pit for the frog to stop. He wouldn't make it. He needed to conserve his strength.

The hope filled frog ignored their warning and jumped even harder. He persisted until, almost miraculously, he got out. Upon reaching the top, the other frogs said, 'We thought there was no way you could jump that high, couldn't you hear us?'

The frog was deaf. He thought they were encouraging and cheering him on the whole time.

Michael, the lesson of this story is that when it comes to your health success, the words of others can greatly impact your attitude and your actions. Ignore the naysayers. Only engage with those who encourage and believe in your ability to succeed. Also, think about what you say to others before speaking to make sure you are being supportive. Because your support can be the difference between their success and their failure."

Michael smiled and spoke. "So, what we choose to hear and think matters."

"Yes," Peale replied. "And so does the voice in your head. Watch your thoughts because they become your words.

Words become actions. Actions become habits. Habits become character. Character becomes destiny."

Just then, Peale gestured toward the shadows. Two wolves stood at the edge of the clearing. One was thin, matted, snarling in circles. The other stood calm, bright-eyed, holding its ground.

"A Cherokee elder once told his grandson that inside us all, two wolves live and fight. One is anger, envy, greed, guilt, and fear. The other is joy, peace, kindness, and faith. Which one wins?"

Michael understood. "The one you feed."

Peale nodded. "You get to choose every day which wolf you are feeding. Are you pouring your energy into resentment and worry, or hope and gratitude?"

Peale placed a glowing key in Michael's hand. It shimmered with shifting hues; the words **Think Positive** and **Rule Eight** etched onto its surface.

"You've got what it takes, Michael. Now believe it."

The city dissolved as Peale's words echoed. The journal opened in Michael's hand. The key's inscription lifted on to the page: **Think Positive. Rule Eight,** and then faded, leaving a gentle warmth.

"Positive thinking isn't pretending problems don't exist.

The power is in not letting them control your mind."

The Eighth Key and Commitment for Health

Think Positive

Today, I choose positive thoughts and forego negative ones. No longer will I be captive to my thoughts.

From now on, I take responsibility for what I allow in my mind. Thoughts are not harmless. They are seeds. What I plant will grow. And what grows shapes my reality, my character, my destiny, my legacy.

I choose to think positively, not as denial of life's difficulties, but to stop letting fear or self-doubt rule me. Life may not always be easy, but I will no longer make it harder by carrying beliefs that drain me.

Every belief I hold was first a thought I repeated. If I want to change my life, I must change my inner language. I will speak to myself with kindness, courage, strength, and possibility.

From now on, I will train my mind like a muscle. I will not focus on defeat or say, "I can't," or "I'm not good enough." Those thoughts are not facts. They are obsolete habits. I now replace them with truth.

I am capable. I am resilient. I am becoming my healthiest self, not by chance, but by choice.

When setbacks come, I won't crumble. I'll reframe, learn, and remember growth comes from challenge. Struggle is not the end, but the start of something greater.

I will surround myself with people who speak positively. I protect my mind from the voices of pessimism and hopelessness. Like the frog in the pit, I'm deaf to discouragement and instead choose to cheer on myself and others.

I accept that every moment is a crossroads. Bitterness or confidence. Anger or gratitude. The wolf that wins is the one I feed. And I choose to feed hope.

I won't wait for proof to believe in my own transformation. Belief is the beginning. I don't need perfection to start thinking better; just a commitment to begin.

I let go of old toxic thoughts and stories that have held me back. I write a new narrative of progress, power, and promise.

From now on, I commit to thinking positive. I'll see setbacks as learning opportunities, find the lesson in storms, and remind myself; I am becoming who I was meant to be.

My commitment is to obey Nature's eighth rule for my health. To think positive. I'll honor it one empowered thought at a time.

Chapter Eleven

Mastering the Circle

Michael stood at the edge of a pier, waves lapping gently below. Fog hung in the early morning air like a woolen shawl, thick and heavy, obscuring the horizon. The scent of salt, fish, and faded burnt wood filled his lungs. In the distance, seagulls called out as if announcing someone's arrival.

He rubbed his eyes, confused. Just moments ago, he'd been sitting at his desk staring at a never-ending stream of unread emails. Now, he was dressed in workout clothes, sneakers damp from the mist.

Behind him, a large brick building loomed, part gym, part fortress. A weather-worn sign hung above the entrance:

Jack LaLanne Physical Culture Studio—Strength Begins Here

Michael turned as the front door creaked open.

A man emerged, broad-shouldered, and impossibly vibrant for his apparent age. His posture was perfect, his handshake firm. Wearing a close-fitting custom jumpsuit and a confident grin, the man had a jaw carved from granite and eyes that sparkled with life.

"You must be Michael," he said.

Michael smiled, "And you are...?"

"Jack LaLanne," he replied with a nod. "Welcome to my world."

Michael had heard of him, of course. The Godfather of Fitness. The man who once swam handcuffed towing boats. The original health evangelist, before wellness was an industry.

Jack turned and motioned him inside.

"Come on. You look like you could use a good sweat and maybe a better perspective."

Inside, the gym hummed with an old-school energy. No flashing screens, no robotic machines. Just iron weights, ropes, mats, medicine balls, and the kind of air that smelled like effort, sweat, and willpower.

Michael followed Jack past a wall of vintage black-and-white photos. There were snapshots of Jack doing one-arm push-ups, pulling airplanes, leaping across rooftops, grinning like a kid who never got tired of being alive.

"You know," Jack said, grabbing a jump rope and tossing another to Michael, "the problem with most people isn't lack of knowledge. It's lack of consistency. You can know everything in the world about being healthy, but if you don't act on it, what good is it?"

Michael caught the rope. "I try. I really do. I start strong and then... life happens."

Jack started jumping in place with graceful ease. "Life's always gonna happen, kid. That's no reason to stop. That's the reason to keep going."

Michael began mimicking the motion, stumbling through the first few rotations.

Jack smiled. "Don't try to be perfect. Just show up."

After a few minutes, Jack motioned to a padded mat in the corner of the gym. They both sat down.

"Today, you are playing the role of Zorro," Jack said, toweling off. "And I'm playing the role of Don Diego."

Michael raised an eyebrow. "Zorro, the masked swordsman?"

"The very one," Jack nodded. "Before he became a legend, Zorro was a mess. He drank too much, was impulsive, emotional, and reckless. Sound familiar?"

Michael smirked. "You've been watching me?"

"I don't have to. Human nature is pretty consistent."

Jack continued. "Zorro wanted to become a master swordsman. He lacked control. So, his mentor, Don Diego, drew a small circle in the dirt, just big enough for Zorro to stand in. He told him, 'You stay in this circle. You move with precision and master every inch of it before you're allowed to move outside. This is your world now.'"

Michael leaned forward, intrigued.

"For days, weeks, Zorro trained in that tiny space. At first, it felt like confinement. Slowly, it became his sanctuary. His skills sharpened. His mind calmed. Only when he mastered that little circle was he allowed to expand his world."

Jack looked Michael straight in the eyes. "That's the key. You want to overhaul everything all at once. Transformation doesn't happen overnight. It happens with seemingly inconsequential changes done consistently over time."

Michael leaned back on his hands, staring at the ceiling beams. "That's easy for you to say. You're built like a superhero. I get winded climbing up stairs."

"Then start with a few stairs at a time. Maybe one flight. Do it again tomorrow. And the next day."

"So, no cape, no gym membership?"

"No cape required. No fancy gyms. Your body and mindset are the only equipment you'll need. Start small. Start with a five-minute walk. One push-up. One glass of water. One less soda. That's your circle."

"Sounds like my to-do list?"

"And you repeat it. Daily. That's where a habit is born. A daily behavior turns into a routine. A routine turns into a habit. A habit then becomes a ritual. You didn't gain weight and become out of shape overnight; what makes you think you can fix it all overnight?"

Michael stood, slowly pacing. "So, how do I stick with it when I don't see immediate results?"

Jack threw him a resistance band. "By focusing on what you can control. You don't need motivation. You need momentum. Let the circle be your starting point. Show up to it every day, and when it becomes second nature, then you expand it. Start with small manageable changes. Progress, not perfection, my friend."

Michael stretched the band, feeling the tension pull across his chest.

Jack walked beside him now. "People want the magic bullet. But here's the truth. Stack little wins. The body responds to consistency, not just intensity."

He stopped in front of a mirror.

"Look at yourself," he said.

Michael glanced up.

"You've got more potential than you give yourself credit for. You've just forgotten how to trust the process."

Jack reached into his pocket and withdrew a key unlike any Michael had ever seen. Shaped like a miniature dumbbell, it carried the weight not only of metal but of purpose. A fine veil of dust clung to its surface, as if it had slumbered for decades, waiting for the right hands to claim it. The metal seemed to hum faintly, catching the light in ripples as Jack turned it. At each rounded end, two concentric rings gleamed, perfectly etched, their edges impossibly precise.

Within the smallest circle, the words *Start Here* were engraved in a script that shimmered like sunlight dancing on water. Encircling it, on the outer ring, the message read: *Rule Nine—Move Your Body Daily.*

As Michael took it, the key felt warm, alive, as though it recognized him. In its weight he sensed movement, rhythm, and the promise of momentum. An unspoken command to awaken not only his body, but his life.

Michael looked at the key with intensity.

"Movement isn't punishment," Jack said. "It's life. The moment you stop moving, you start aging. The less you move, the stiffer you get. The stiffer you get, the less you move. It's a vicious downward spiral."

They walked outside, the fog now lifting as the sun broke through. Waves danced under the growing light. Jack pointed at a nearby pier rail. "Every day, I start by doing one thing for my body before I do anything for the world. It doesn't have to be flashy. Just has to be mine."

Michael looked out over the water. "So, the secret is... don't try to change everything. Just win the circle."

"Exactly," Jack said. "Do five push-ups. Make it so small you can't fail."

"Five push-ups, huh? What if I collapse after two?"

"Then tomorrow you go for three. Expand the circle only when you master it."

He placed a hand on Michael's shoulder. "Promise me this: Never let another day pass where you ignore your own health for the sake of a to-do list. Because if you don't have your health, you can't show up for any of it."

Michael nodded, the breeze cooling the sweat on his skin. "I think I'm ready to start."

"Good," Jack smiled. "Just remember, no more guilt. No more all-or-nothing. Just small wins repeated daily. That's how we turn the impossible into inevitable."

Jack turned and walked away. As Jack's figure faded from view, Michael stood holding the dumbbell-shaped key, *Start Here. Rule Nine—Move Your Body Daily.* The words seemed to pulse faintly, as if each beat carried the rhythm of a heartbeat in motion. He opened the journal, its pages alive with quiet anticipation.

Guided by the same instinct that had merged the earlier keys, he set the dumbbell key across the open page. At once, a deep golden light began to spill from its surface, flowing like molten sunlight into the paper's fibers. The concentric rings on the key's ends began to spin slowly, not mechanically, but like small waves moving outward across still water.

The inner circle's engraving, *Start Here* lifted from the metal as threads of light, drifting down onto the page. Then the outer ring's inscription, *Rule Nine—Move Your Body Daily*, followed, its letters unfurling into the paper like roots sinking deep into soil. The key's shape dissolved next, breaking into radiant fragments that sank into the journal until no trace remained.

When Michael ran his fingertips over the spot, the page felt warm, almost breathing, and he could swear he felt a subtle vibration, like the steady, reassuring rhythm of footsteps on a long road ahead.

> Don't try to change everything.
>
> Just win the circle.

The Ninth Key and Commitment for Health

Move Your Body Daily

Today, I will honor my body with movement. I will move and do physical activity for overall health and fitness.

I will no longer see exercise and physical activity as a chore. I will no longer wait for motivation to appear. I understand now that movement is a gift, not a task. It is a privilege, not a punishment.

From this moment forward, I will move my body every day, with gratitude, deliberately, joyfully, consistently. Not because I have to, simply because I can.

I will stop searching for the perfect workout or waiting for the perfect moment. I will no longer attempt to do everything at once, only to do nothing at all. Now I know the secret: I will start small and stay consistent. I will master the circle I am in before moving to the larger one.

A short walk, a few stretches, a dance in my kitchen, a climb up the stairs. These are not trivial acts. These are triumphs. These are choices that build momentum, confidence, and health from the inside out.

I will stop believing the lie that I must suffer to make progress. I will no longer associate movement with guilt, shame, or regret. I move to celebrate life, not escape it.

I accept that strength is built, not wished for. Energy is earned, not bought. I will move daily because my body was made for motion, not stagnation. My muscles crave engagement. My heart longs for rhythm. My mind clears when I move with intention.

From this day forward, I commit to do as much physical activity daily as possible. I will not compare my pace to anyone else's. I will not let perfection rob me of progress. Every step, every rep, every stretch is a victory.

I will make movement a ritual, not a reaction. I will protect it on my calendar and honor it like a sacred meeting with my future self. Because every time I move, I remind myself that I am not stuck. I am in motion, becoming stronger, healthier, and more alive.

My commitment is to obey Nature's ninth rule to move and do physical activities daily for my health. And I will honor it one step at a time.

Chapter Twelve

The Return

The sterile scent of antiseptic lingered in the air, sharp and cold. Beeping monitors pulsed, echoing like distant memories. Michael's eyelids fluttered open, heavy with confusion.

Fluorescent lights cast a white glow above, making him squint. The rhythmic whoosh of an oxygen machine filled the space. Everything felt muted, as if wrapped in gauze.

He turned his head. The stiff pillow crinkled beneath it. Beside him sat Sarah, her eyes rimmed red, now full of relief. Her hand clutched his.

"You're awake," she whispered, brushing a stray hair from her face. "Oh, thank God, Michael. You scared us."

His voice, hoarse and rough, squeaked, "What... what happened?"

She exhaled, her voice gentle but trembling. "You passed out. Right in the middle of Emily's piano recital. One moment you were next to me, clapping and the next you slumped over. They think it was due to exhaustion, stress, high blood pressure. You might be diabetic. They're still running tests."

Emily. The recital. It returned, flooding in; his daughter's small fingers poised on the piano keys, the room filled with proud parents, the scent of polished wood and stage lights. Then... darkness.

"I..." He trailed off. The memories from the past day or had it been weeks? Just dreams? Echoes lingered in his bones.

Sarah cupped his face, tears streaming down her pale face. She couldn't hide her red eyes. "You've been out almost twenty-four hours. Michael, I thought I lost you."

She wiped her eyes and continued, "Emily's with your sister. She didn't want to leave your side, but the doctors thought it was best. They almost put you into an induced coma until they figured out what was wrong.

"Michael, the doctor said you're going to need to make some major lifestyle changes. No more skipped meals. No more fourteen-hour days. No more energy drinks. We need you. I need you."

Her words struck him, not as guilt, but as grace. She kissed his forehead and stepped out to talk to the nurse, promising to be right back.

Left alone, Michael lay still. A slow realization rose through the fog: the mentors, the journal, the keys. Had it all been a dream? Something had shifted inside, something that no brain scan or medical test could explain.

He slowly rolled onto his side and reached for the folded pants on the chair. He grimaced with pain but did not stop. His fingers fumbled in the pocket.

He found it. Soft, familiar, undeniably real.

His heart pounded as he pulled out a small, leather-bound journal, worn at the edges yet impossibly pristine. He opened it to the first page. As he flipped through the pages, radiant gold ink shimmered under the hospital light, words that had appeared after each encounter on his journey.

Rule One: Drink more water. It's the simplest act of self-respect.

Rule Two: Refuse sugar and ultra-processed foods.

Rule Three: Eat real, holistic, whole foods.

Rule Four: Eat slowly and mindfully.

Rule Five: Eat small portions.

Rule Six: Get adequate sleep.

Rule Seven: Rest to digest.

Rule Eight: Think positive.

Rule Nine: Move daily.

Rule Ten: Share the journey. He wasn't sure if his mind just forgot this one or if he had more to learn.

Each page glowed with its own truth etched into the parchment like commandments from another realm. His fingers traced the pages; a chill ran through him.

It had all been real.

The monk, the summit, the banquet. Adelle Davis's wisdom, Jack LaLanne's firm grip, Halbert Dunn's encouragement, Hippocrates' fierce gaze, Paul Bragg's quiet strength, and the others, too.

The mentors hadn't just taught him; they'd awakened a knowing. The path forward was no longer theory. It existed.

Except, Rule Ten. There was no mentor for the tenth rule.

That's odd, he thought.

Tears welled, not from sorrow, but deep gratitude.

His fingertips brushed the pocket seam of his pants, noticing a subtle bulge. Curious, he pulled out something cool and solid.

A key, unlike any other, a delicate circle at the bow with two figures walking side by side on a winding path that disappeared into the horizon. Etched along the shaft: **Share the Journey**. On the reverse, graceful script: **Rule Ten**.

The key felt warm, as if it had been carried by countless hands. Michael knew instantly it was more than a key. It was an invitation.

Drawn by instinct, he placed it on the journal. For a moment, nothing happened. Then, as soft golden light seeped from the key, flowing like water into the cover. The carved figures shimmered, blurring into a thread of light before melting away. The faint impression left behind seemed as if it had always belonged.

Tracing it with his fingers, Michael felt a subtle pulse, alive and waiting. He could sense the journal would open to a new entry when the time was right. For now, one message was clear:

No one climbs alone. No one heals alone. Share the journey, and the road will rise to meet you.

As Sarah returned, Michael flipped to the final page. There, in bold script it said:

The Tenth Key: Share the Journey

Health isn't a destination. It's a journey. And this journey creates a ripple, like a stone cast into a small pond. The path was never meant to be walked alone.

You don't fully own your transformation until you share your knowledge with others. Don't hoard health like a secret recipe. Be a beacon, show the way with sensitivity, sincerity, empathy, authenticity, and quiet strength.

When others see your energy, your clarity, your renewed presence... they'll ask, What changed?

That's your cue to begin.

Share what you've learned. Not to preach, not to impress, but to invite. Health is contagious when shared with love. Someone you care about is still struggling. Your story may be the lifeline they never knew they needed.

Michael exhaled.

The machine's beeps marked time. Nurses' quiet steps passed by. Down the hall, a laugh echoed. Life was moving, waiting for Michael to catch up.

He pressed the journal to his chest, closed his eyes, and let the truth settle in.

He had been given a second chance. A new path to follow.

This time, he wouldn't stray.

> No one climbs alone. No one heals alone.
>
> Share the journey and the road will rise to meet you.

Chapter Thirteen

A New Beginning

Michael stepped out of the hospital's sliding doors into the warm sunlight. Billowing clouds scattered across a vivid blue sky. The air felt different, crisper, brighter. For the first time in years, he wasn't glued to his phone or mentally scrolling through unread emails. He was, simply, breathing.

Sarah stood by his side, her arm through his, while Emily skipped ahead on the sidewalk. Michael smiled. The beeping monitors, sterile walls, and doctor's warnings had left a permanent mark; not of fear, but resolve. He vowed never to return to the life that broke him.

At home, Michael sat quietly at his desk, the journal open before him. The last key imprint still warm in his palm. The air felt charged. Not with sound or movement, but with the sense that something exceptional was about to happen.

He stroked the journal's cover. The leather felt dense, alive. The hum he'd felt after each key merged with the pages was now a steady vibration beneath his fingertips. Suddenly, the journal stirred.

Light seeped from its seams, a soft gold at first, joined by threads of blue, green, rose, and silver. They were the colors of the keys, of the lessons, of every moment he'd earned.

One by one, engravings appeared: Drink Pure Water. Refuse Refined Sugar and Ultra-Processed Foods. Eat Real Food. Eat Slowly and Mindfully. Eat Small Portions. Sleep/Healthy Sleep. Rest to Digest. Think Positive. Move Your Body Daily. Share the Journey. Each glowed, its rhythm matching his heartbeat.

The symbols connected. Light streaming between them like constellations. The vibration deepened through his chest until it reached his bones.

The pages fluttered open on their own, stopping at the very first blank sheet. In luminous script: **All keys found. The door is ready.**

A stillness fell. Michael sensed the energy was no longer on the page, it was inside him now. The warmth, the colors, and pulse were part of him, as if the journal had been waiting to return the keys to their true home.

He closed the journal gently. It no longer felt like a book, but a living record of who he had become and a promise of who he would continue to be.

Within two months, Michael made the decision he once thought unthinkable. He sold his business, not for the highest offer, but to the buyer who promised to preserve the culture and take care of his employees. "You could've gotten double," people said.

"I got something more valuable. Freedom and time," he replied.

No longer trapped in the rat race, he chose to live, not just exist.

With newfound freedom, Michael built a new rhythm. Mornings started with a walk in the park, water bottle in hand. Lunches were light and mindful. Dinners around the table, no TV, no rushing. He went to bed earlier, read more, laughed more. He rebuilt his life, one key at a time.

His story wasn't just for him.

Invitations began trickling in from friends, colleagues, and eventually business groups who noticed his transformation. One financial advisor asked Michael to speak to his clients about "how to protect the most important asset: your health." The response was electric. Conference rooms filled with people who had everything except energy and joy.

Michael's calendar filled: wellness workshops, keynote talks, community events. He stood before exhausted executives, stressed parents, and burned-out teams, sharing the Ten Keys, the path he'd found in that old leather journal.

Then came LIFE 42 Wellness. For Michael, LIFE 42 Wellness felt like the missing piece. It wasn't a program that demanded perfection or another fad that promised results and left people disappointed. Instead, it gave a clear path with simple daily actions that fit into life without being overwhelming. He surrounded himself with others walking the same road, held them accountable, offered encouragement, and shared the lessons from his mentors.

He wasn't just living his second chance. He was echoing it.

> "The Keys are now yours.
>
> What you choose to do with them is up to you."

Chapter Fourteen

Days of Future Past

Stella Point, Tanzania, Africa, 4:30 a.m.

The world was silent and dark, except for the crunch of boots against volcanic gravel and scree; the rasp of heavy breaths drawn from the frozen air. Michael Caldwell stood at Stella Point, 18,885 feet above sea level, the lower summit of Mount Kilimanjaro. Wind howled like a ghost across the crater rim, cutting through even the thickest silence. Overhead, the stars flickered like distant memories, and the horizon far to the east whispered hints of dawn.

Michael pulled his parka zipper all the way up, burying his face beneath layers of insulation. Frost crusted at the seams of his goggles. Each exhale fogged the air before vanishing into the void. A wool beanie hugged his head beneath his hood, and his glacier-grade gloves were stiff and clumsy, but necessary. Every inch of skin was covered, but the cold cut through him like a knife.

Beside him, Robert Perkins, a longtime friend of Michael's, exhaled heavily, and adjusted the strap on his pack. His cheeks were ruddy; his beard crusted with ice. Yet despite the surroundings, his eyes sparkled.

"You remember ten years ago?" Robert asked, his voice muffled under his thermal buff. "When you told me you'd never do this. That you hated the cold. Hated hiking."

Michael managed a chuckle, more a grunt in the high altitude. "I also said I'd never drink protein smoothies. Never sell the business. Never become a journaling guy. Shows what I knew."

Robert leaned on his trekking pole, laughing. "You were stubborn as hell back then. Still are. But when you finally walked away from Caldwell & Associates... everything changed."

Michael nodded, his eyes fixed ahead. Even in the dark, he could make out the faint silhouette of Uhuru Peak, the highest point on the continent. It was a brutal incline that still lay ahead.

"I held onto that company like a lifeline," Michael admitted. "Thought if I let go, I'd drown in regret."

"And?"

"I didn't drown," Michael said, voice soft. "I floated. I found my breath again."

Robert grinned, lines deepening in his wind-burned face. "I'll never forget when you called and said you were down thirty pounds, off the blood pressure meds, hiking local trails like a madman."

Michael flexed his gloved hands and rolled his shoulders. "It wasn't just the weight. It was like taking off a suit of armor I'd worn for decades. When I sold the company, joined LIFE 42, started mentoring others... this trip became the exclamation point. The reward."

They stood quietly, the wind whispering around them.

Robert smiled beneath his frostbitten cheeks. "Let's get to Uhuru Peak before the sun does."

They began the final ascent. A line of headlamps danced both above and below. The world was silent, but for the crunch of boots and the whip of the mountain wind. Uhuru (Swahili for freedom) was within reach.

Uhuru Peak—5:45 a.m.

The last push from Stella Point to Uhuru Peak was less than an hour, but at nearly 19,400 feet above sea level, where time lost all meaning. Each step felt like trudging through wet cement in a snowstorm. Michael forced himself to count to ten between steps, plant a foot, then the next, breathe, rest, repeat.

Through the half-light, the summit sign appeared at last, wooden and weathered, ringed in frost. A few other climbers clustered nearby, their down parkas vivid against the vast snow. In their triumph, most looked dazed, leaning on their poles or huddling in hoods. Some wept quietly. Others simply stared in awe and exhaustion.

The thin, icy wind stung Michael's cheeks. But inside he was glowing.

"Almost there," Robert rasped, breath white and shallow.

Their pace slowed even further. Michael blinked through the goggles as tears pricked his eyes, part cold, part disbelief. Nothing, no photo, no documentary, no tale from a friend, could prepare him for this moment.

Their guide, Steven, nodded, motioning their group for photos. "You, next, my friends," the guide said.

Michael and Robert stepped up to the summit sign together. The sun was just beginning to rise.

The full text etched in bright yellow on the old wooden planks read:

"Mount Kilimanjaro Congratulations! You are now at Uhuru Peak, Tanzania, 5895M/19341ft AMSL. Africa's Highest Point. World's Highest Free-Standing Mountain."

Michael stood in awe while the sky turned orange and gold, casting light over the glaciers flanking the peak. Their group handed over cameras and posed quickly, then raised their trekking poles like swords, arms linked.

Quiet celebration, too tired for words.

But Michael didn't care.

His heart thundered not from exertion, but exhilaration.

He stepped back, giving the next climbers their turn, then stood at the edge of the crater rim. Below, the glaciers shimmered like ancient sentinels. The sun inched above the horizon, spilling golden light.

Robert stepped up beside him, breathless. "You did it, Mike."

Michael shook his head slowly, watching the sunrise. "No," he whispered, "We did it."

He slipped off a glove, reaching into his parka pocket, and pulled out the journal he had carried since that past life. His transformation lived in simple things: the magical keys etched on the worn cover from years of use.

He held the journal in his bare palm, watching the light glint off the keys' golden images.

Around them, the group gathered, hugs, smiles through frozen lashes, exchanging quiet congratulations.

Michael approached the summit marker. He pressed his gloved hand to the frost-covered wood and whispered a simple prayer of thanks.

This mountain hasn't been conquered. It has been revealed.

Uhuru. Freedom. Not from responsibility, but from the weight of who he had been. He felt lighter, not just in body, but in spirit.

The descent began almost immediately after reaching the summit. Michael was not the same man who had started the climb.

The Descent—Barafu Base Camp

As they descended from Uhuru Peak, the air felt heavier, warmer. The adrenaline still faintly pulsed through him even though exhaustion set in. The sun bleached the glacier fields, and the ice was treacherous.

The group trekked quietly, poles clacking against volcanic rock. The journey down was fast, but cautious, each step a drop in altitude, each breath a touch easier. Total focus was needed.

Michael's thighs trembled, knees ached, sweat pooled inside his gloves. But he was steady. What had taken days to climb, they descended in hours.

They finally reached Barafu Base Camp, at 15,331 feet, feeling as if they arrived on another planet. Tents dotted the slope like colorful beetles. Porters greeted them with warm ginger tea and applause. But most only smiled faintly or nodded, before crawling into tents for sleep.

Michael unzipped his pack, groaned as he pulled off his boots and collapsed into his sleeping bag.

He slept for just under two hours, just enough.

By mid-morning, their group gathered again, boots laced. The trail to Mweka Camp for lunch became an alpine meadow. Gone were the icy ridges and howling wind.

The trip moved quickly. No one needed to talk. Each step held quiet reflection. The trail twisted through rocks and trees. Porters sped ahead hurrying home. Michael admired their speed and strength.

Eventually, they reached the exit at Mweka Gate. After signing out and receiving certificates beneath an overhang, they found lunch: hot stew, fried bananas, rice, vegetables, and fresh mango juice. Someone joked, "Anyone want to do this again?" Almost in unison the response was, "Hell no." The camaraderie was unspoken yet deeply felt.

Michael ate slowly, savoring each bite. His body ached, but his spirit soared. He scribbled in his journal not wanting to forget the climb, the descent, the lessons carved deeper than ever.

They browsed the souvenir stands. Beadwork, carvings, and paintings. Michael bought a simple bracelet for Emily, a blue Tanzanite for Sarah, and a black and white painting of a rhinoceros for himself. It wasn't about the souvenirs; it was the experience, the memories that would live within him.

He looked back one last time at the peak, still cloaked in clouds. He realized that the real summit wasn't up there, it was ahead, wherever the next step led.

Chapter Fifteen

Echolitus

There is a condition I started calling Echolitus.

You won't find it in any medical journal. No doctor will diagnose it. No prescription will treat it. But you have it. So does almost everyone you know. And it is killing more people slowly than most of the diseases that make the news.

Echolitus is what happens when the messages we hear about food become louder than the signals our own bodies send. It is the slow accumulation of marketing echoes in the mind until the echoes feel like truth, and the truth feels like noise.

We didn't choose this. We were born into it. From the moment we could understand language, we were taught what to crave, what to trust, and what to call healthy. Not by our grandmothers in their kitchens. Not by farmers at the market. By food companies who spent billions of dollars learning exactly how to make us listen.

Look at the words stamped on the front of the packages: Low-fat. Heart-healthy. Natural. Guilt-free. Fuel your day. Snack smart.

These phrases echo through grocery aisles, television commercials, social media feeds, and packaging designed to make poison look like nourishment. Repeat anything often enough and the brain stops questioning it. That's not weakness. That's biology. The human mind is built to trust what it hears often. The food industry knows this better than we do.

The result is a population that cannot remember what real hunger feels like, what real food tastes like, or what a body that runs on actual nourishment feels like in the morning.

Michael had been living with Echolitus for thirty years before he had a name for it.

The pull toward the energy drink at three in the afternoon—that was Echolitus. The belief that a granola bar marked "wholesome" was a healthy breakfast—that was Echolitus. The conviction that he was too busy to cook, too tired to plan, too far gone to change—those were echoes too. Not his thoughts. Not really. They were repeated messages he had absorbed so deeply they felt like his own voice.

You may recognize the signs in yourself.

Persistent weight that no diet seems to resolve. Cravings that arrive on schedule, triggered not by hunger but by a commercial, a smell, a brightly colored package at a checkout counter. Afternoon crashes that you treat with sugar or caffeine, which lead to evening crashes that you treat with comfort food, which lead to mornings that begin with confusion about what to eat. A vague guilt about food that never quite goes away, no matter how careful you try to be.

This is not a personal failure. This is what happens when an entire culture has been trained over generations to mistake engineered products for nourishment.

The food industry calls it consumer behavior. The medical industry calls it lifestyle disease. I call it Echolitus, because naming a thing is the first step in seeing it.

And once you see it, you cannot unsee it.

You walk into a grocery store and notice that the packages are designed to look healthy. You read an ingredient list and recognize chemistry rather than food. You hear a slogan and feel the small click of recognition: *that is an echo, not a truth.* You begin to ask different questions. Not "what should I eat?" but "who is telling me what to eat, and what do they gain by my listening?"

The recovery from Echolitus is not a diet. It is not a program. It is not another set of rules to follow until you fail.

The recovery is remembering.

Remembering that your grandmother knew how to cook without a label telling her what was healthy. Remembering that real food does not need to advertise itself. Remembering that your body sends signals—true hunger, true thirst, true fatigue, true satiety—and that those signals were drowned out by the echoes, not by your character.

The path back is not loud. It is quieter than the world that made you sick. It is one glass of water before coffee. One whole food on the plate instead of a packaged product. One question asked before a craving is obeyed: *am I hungry, or am I echoing?*

When you stop listening to the echoes and start listening to your body, health returns. Not all at once. Not dramatically. But steadily, the way trees grow and tides shift and seeds become trees.

The cure for Echolitus is not punishment or restriction. It is not guilt, shame, or another impossible promise in a glossy wrapper.

The cure is remembering. Listening. Rebuilding a relationship with nourishment the way one rebuilds faith—gently, patiently, truthfully.

Michael had been deaf to his body for thirty years. The mentors he met on his journey were not teaching him new information. They were teaching him to hear what had been there all along.

The echoes do not have to win. Not in your life. Not in your family. Not in the next generation.

Once you can name the condition, you have already begun to heal.

> Health doesn't come from what others tell you.
>
> It comes from what you finally decide to tell yourself.

Welcome to LIFE 42 Wellness

You only get one body. Let's make it count because your health can't wait. Here's your invitation to reset your health and lifestyle.

If you're holding this book, chances are you've felt that quiet whisper in the back of your mind:

I can't keep living like this.

The fatigue. The brain fog. The stress eating. The scale creeping up. The prescription bottles piling up. Even worse... the slow loss of your spark.

We get it because we've been there. We found a path forward that delivers real results.

Welcome to **LIFE 42 Wellness**, a space where real people reclaim their energy, confidence, and health, doing seven simple tasks, one day at a time.

This isn't another fad. It's not about calorie counting or willpower. It's not about chasing a number on a scale.

It's about healing.

Because weight loss isn't the goal. It's a natural side effect of healing your body from the inside out.

LIFE 42 is built around a proven, science-backed recipe:

42 days. 7 daily actions. 1 commitment... to yourself.

Inside LIFE 42, you'll get:

- **Clarity**—You will know exactly what to do every day. No guesswork.
- **Accountability**—You're not alone. We walk with you.
- **Support**—A real community that lifts you when you stumble. Individual and group coaching.
- **Momentum**—From day one, you'll feel it: more energy, fewer cravings, deeper sleep, stronger habits.

And the best part?

- It's not a quick fix—**it's a lifestyle you grow into.**
- It's not expensive—it's intentionally designed to be affordable for anyone who's ready to invest in their health.
- It's not complicated—just 7 small simple and easy tasks each day that stack into lifelong change.

You don't need more willpower. You need direction, a plan that fits real life, and people in your corner.

Here's what we believe:

- Health isn't about being perfect.
- It's not about doing more.
- It's about doing what matters, consistently.

If you've tried everything and nothing stuck...

If you're tired of starting over...

If you want to feel *alive* again...

This is your second chance. Not next week. Not next year. **Right now.**

Let this be your moment. The moment you say:

I'm ready. I'm worth it. I will not settle for anything less than a life I love living.

Join LIFE 42 Wellness and take your first step toward healing, energy, and confidence.

https://life42.ai

> Prevention is always better than a health crisis.
>
> Your health won't wait. Neither should you.

The Ten Keys And Commitments For Living A Vibrant, Healthy Life

First Key

Drink Pure Water

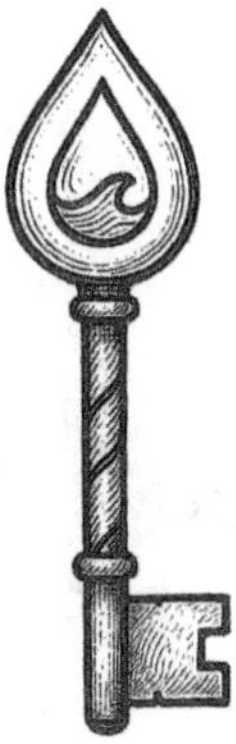

The first and most essential commitment to health is drinking pure water. I resolve to honor my body by choosing water as my primary source of nourishment, no longer ignoring the truth that my body depends on it for clarity, energy, and vitality. I reject sodas, energy drinks, sugary teas, and artificially colored beverages, acknowledging that my mind's fog and body's aches are warnings I can no longer ignore.

I accept responsibility for my own health, not delegating it to doctors or medicine, and make drinking pure water daily an intentional act of self-care. Carrying a water bottle will serve as a symbol of my commitment to a healthy lifestyle. Water reminds me that I am worthy of care and can always begin again. I let go of the belief that hydration requires flavor or is difficult; water is simple, sacred, and essential.

By choosing water, I choose clarity, energy, and healing. I act now, not waiting for illness to motivate me, and embrace prevention, nourishment, and life itself. From this day forward, I commit to drinking pure water as the foundation of my wellness, refusing to let dehydration diminish my well-being. In doing so, I honor the natural law of staying hydrated, one sip at a time.

The Second Key and Commitment for Health

Refuse Refined Sugar

Today, I reclaim my power by rejecting the false promise of sugar, which offers comfort but ultimately steals energy, clouds my mind, and weakens my resolve. I am no longer deceived by sweet cravings or manipulated by processed foods; my decision to avoid refined sugar is not about deprivation but about freedom and self-empowerment.

I recognize sugar's addictive nature and refuse to surrender my health for momentary pleasure or convenience. By saying "no" to sugar, I say "yes" to clarity, stability, and sustained energy. I no longer allow my moods, energy, or health to be dictated by sugary treats or manufactured foods.

While resisting sugar may be uncomfortable at first, I know my body and taste buds will adapt, and my overall well-being will improve. I do not need a diagnosis or a doctor's permission to make this change; I accept that sugar contributes to inflammation, weight gain, and chronic disease, and I choose to act now before regret.

This commitment is not about perfection but about progress and creating a healthier future for myself. From this day forward, I avoid refined sugar and highly processed foods, honoring my body with nourishing choices and respecting Nature's law, one decision at a time.

The Third Key and Commitment for Health

Eat Real Food

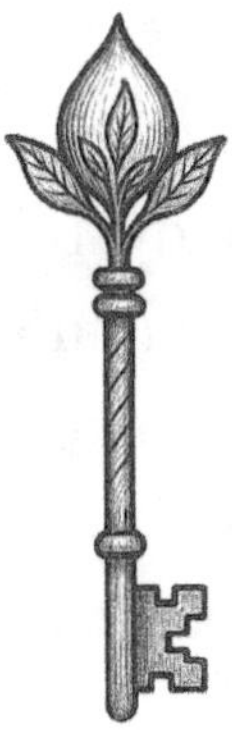

Today, I choose to nourish my body with the raw materials nature intended, recognizing that food is fuel and the foundation of my well-being. From now on, I commit to eating whole, unprocessed foods, those that grow in the ground, swim in the sea, or walk the earth, free from artificial additives or factory modifications.

I will not be fooled by convenience, packaging, or marketing claims. I understand there is a difference between foods that simply fill me and those that truly nourish and heal my body. Food is not entertainment, a reward, or a remedy for emotional discomfort; it is a sacred exchange between earth and body, deserving of respect.

I will question the origins and quality of what I eat, seeking foods as close to their natural state as possible, and rejecting those altered to enhance shelf life or appeal. My commitment is to build my body with care, using the best ingredients, understanding that every bite is either supporting or undermining my health.

While I strive for progress, not perfection, I accept that setbacks may happen and will use each day as a new opportunity to make better choices. I forgive past mistakes and now honor my body with nutritious, real food, committing to feed my health and uphold Nature's third rule, one mindful bite at a time.

The Fourth Key and Commitment for Health

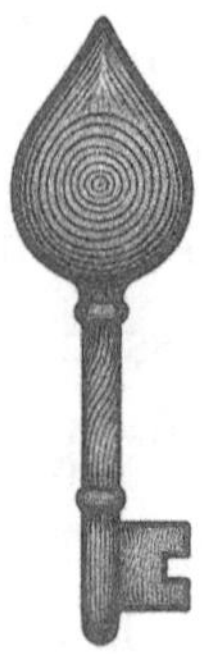

Eat Slowly and Mindfully

Today, I honor my body by being fully present with my meals, no longer rushing through eating or making it an afterthought. I now understand that how, when, and what I eat are all equally important.

From this day forward, I commit to eating with gratitude and intention—without distractions like screens or cars, and not out of habit or stress. I will slow down, chew intentionally, and truly taste my food. Each bite becomes an opportunity to connect with my body and invite healing.

I will not use food to numb emotions or escape discomfort. Instead, I will listen to my body's true needs, distinguishing between hunger, thirst, rest, and emotional cravings. I release the notion that eating more means greater satisfaction, committing instead to eat until I am nourished, not numb.

Meals are not interruptions but sacred pauses, moments to reconnect, express gratitude, and be present. Though mindful eating may feel awkward at first, it is an act of respect for my body and a way to cultivate a healthy relationship with food.

I forgive past mistakes and rushed meals, choosing instead to honor my body with attention and care. Mindful eating isn't about strict rules, but about respecting the body's needs and the food that sustains it. By slowing down and paying attention, I foster healing and nourishment.

From now on, I will savor my meals, honor the sources and preparation of my food, and nurture my body, one conscious bite at a time, in alignment with Nature's fourth rule for health.

The Fifth Key and Commitment for Health

Eat Small Portions

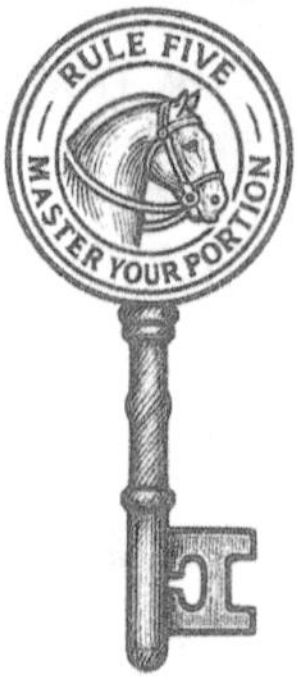

Today, I choose to honor my body by focusing on quality over quantity, no longer confusing indulgence with nourishment. I commit to eating small portions deliberately and mindfully, nourishing myself to thrive rather than to numb.

I let go of the myth that more food means greater satisfaction or fulfillment. I trust my body to signal when it's had enough and view hunger as a helpful guide, not an enemy. Portion control, for me, is not about restriction but about respect. Each bite affirms my care and attention to my body's needs.

I intentionally downsize my plate, slow my pace, and eat with full presence. I will no longer use excess food to cope with stress or emotion, nor trade long-term health for momentary gratification.

From this day forward, I commit to mastering my portions, choosing awareness and quality over habit and excess. In doing so, I reclaim clarity, energy, and well-being, honoring Nature's fifth rule for health, one intentional bite at a time.

The Sixth Key and Commitment for Health

Healthy Sleep

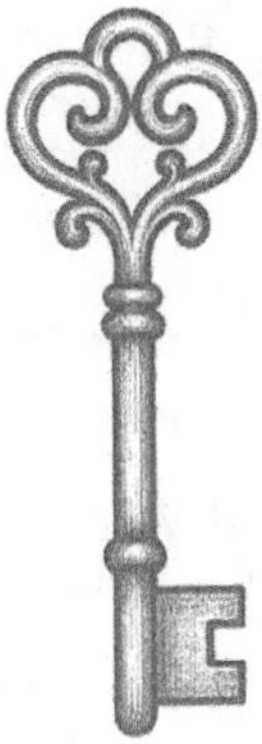

Today, I choose to see rest not as a weakness or a reward, but as a necessity for well-being and restoration. I reject the idea that exhaustion or burnout signifies dedication—fatigue is not productive, and sleep is not wasted time.

From now on, I will prioritize sleep, understanding it as vital for physical repair, mental clarity, and emotional balance. Sleeplessness is not a sign of commitment, but a form of self-neglect. I listen to my body's signals, release the cycle of overwork, and stop chasing goals on empty.

I commit to creating soothing bedtime rituals that promote calm and quality rest. Rest is an act of self-respect and resistance in a culture obsessed with hustle, and I will honor my need for it.

I will not rely on caffeine or adrenaline to push through fatigue. Instead, I embrace the wisdom of my body, allowing it to recover and thrive through adequate sleep. Sleep is a fundamental law of nature, essential for regeneration and overall health.

From today forward, I commit to making sleep a

priority, protecting my rest, and recognizing that when I sleep well, I live well. By honoring sleep, I honor life itself, one sacred night at a time.

The Seventh Key and Commitment for Health

Rest to Digest

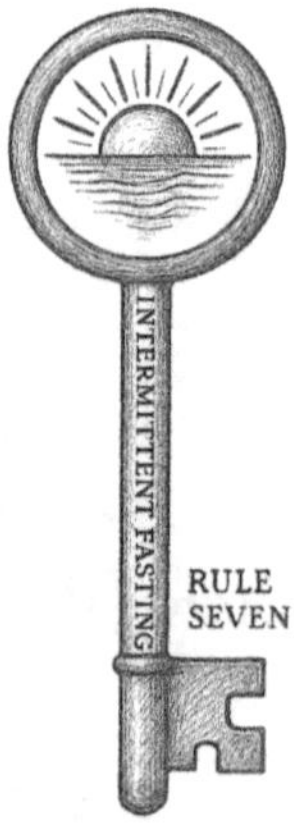

Today, I honor my body's natural rhythms by allowing time for rest, repair, and rejuvenation between meals. I reject the idea of treating my digestive system like a machine made for constant consumption or believing that frequent eating equates to better health.

Instead, I recognize that healing requires pauses and that true nourishment comes from mindful intervals between meals. By allowing my body to fast and rest, I support its natural ability to cleanse, balance, and repair itself. Fasting is not starvation, but a wise structure that helps restore my body's natural cadence.

From now on, I will listen to my body, wait to eat until true hunger returns, and resist the urge to fill every empty space. I will fast overnight and break my fast only when my body is ready, not according to the clock or habit. I will tune out external pressures and cravings, embracing the power of stillness and the clarity, balance, and peace it brings.

This is my commitment to Nature's seventh rule for health: to rest for digestion. I will honor my body's need for space and balance, one intentional pause at a time.

The Eighth Key and Commitment for Health

Think Positive

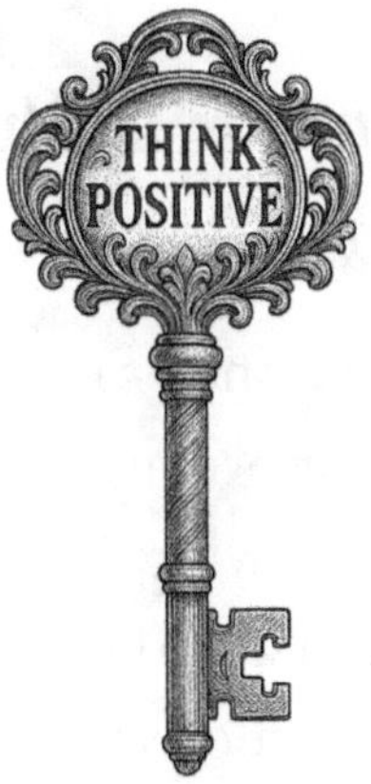

Today, I take responsibility for my thoughts, understanding that what I allow in my mind shapes my reality, character, and destiny. I choose positive thinking, not to ignore life's challenges, but to refuse to let fear and self-doubt control me.

I recognize that beliefs begin as repeated thoughts, so I commit to changing my inner language, replacing negative habits with affirmations of courage, strength, and possibility. I am capable and resilient, and I choose to become my healthiest self by conscious choice, not by chance.

When setbacks arise, I will reframe them as opportunities for growth, viewing struggles as beginnings, not endings. I will surround myself with positive influences and protect my mind from negativity, focusing on hope, gratitude, and encouragement.

Each moment presents a decision: to feed bitterness or confidence, anger or gratitude. Today, I choose to nurture hope and believe in my own transformation, letting go of toxic stories and writing a new narrative of progress and possibility.

From this day forward, I commit to thinking positive, viewing setbacks as learning experiences, and honoring Nature's eighth law for health, one empowered thought at a time.

The Ninth Key and Commitment for Health

Move Your Body Daily

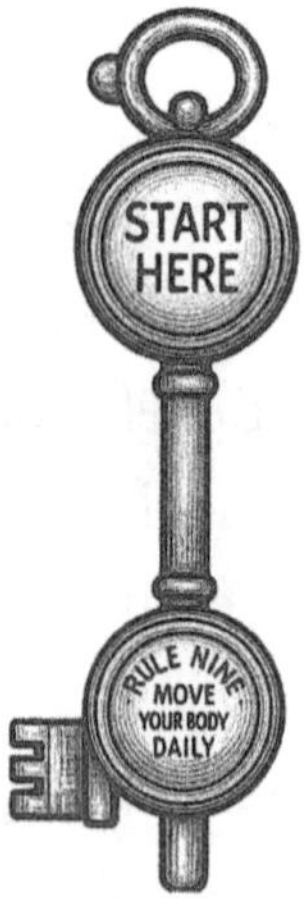

Today, I choose to honor my body through regular movement and physical activity, viewing it as a privilege rather than a chore. I will no longer wait for motivation or perfection; instead, I will start with small, consistent actions performed with gratitude and joy.

Whether it's a walk, stretching, dancing, or climbing stairs, I recognize that every bit of movement contributes to my well-being, building confidence, momentum, and health from within. I reject the idea that progress requires suffering or that movement should be associated with guilt or regret. Instead, I move to celebrate life and support my body's natural need for motion.

I accept that strength and energy are developed over

time through consistent effort, not through comparison or perfectionism. Each step, stretch, or rep is a victory, and making movement a daily ritual keeps me growing, healthy, and full of life.

From this day forward, I commit to daily physical activity, respecting my own pace and progress, and honoring Nature's ninth rule for health—one step at a time.

The Tenth Key and Commitment for Health

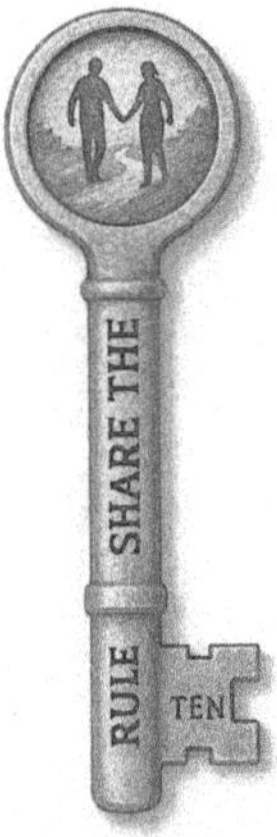

Share the Journey

Health is not a final destination, but an ongoing journey that creates a ripple effect, influencing those around us. True transformation is fully realized when we share it with others, not by preaching or seeking admiration, but by inviting and inspiring with sincerity, empathy, and authenticity.

When people notice your increased energy and clarity, your openness to sharing can become a lifeline for someone in need. Health is contagious when shared with love, and your story may offer hope and guidance to someone still struggling. Be a beacon by sharing your journey, inviting others to join you on the path to wellness.

A Final Word From Michael

If there's one thing my journey has taught me, it's this, sometimes the enemy isn't just in our minds, it's in our pantry.

Years before I collapsed at Emily's recital, the trap had been set. Food scientists were studying my brain, our brains, like interrogators. Every processed snack was engineered to hijack my willpower.

Back in 1999, Frito-Lay hired neuroscientists to find the "bliss point;" the ideal blend of salt, fat, sugar, and texture that keeps you eating "just one more." Once that secret was found, the entire food industry adopted it.

These snacks are not food. They're edible drugs. The industry uses what I call The Addiction Formula:

- Crunchy textures that trigger reward pathways in your brain.
- Vanishing caloric density so you never feel full.

- Hyper-palatable combinations of salt + fat + sugar that make moderation nearly impossible.

They spend billions a year on this science.

And we pay the price with our health, our wallets, and our lives.

This is not a willpower problem. It's biology.

Both processed food and drugs light up the same brain parts. Both create tolerance, more for the same effect. Both cause withdrawal when you try to quit.

I lived it. I broke free.

If you want out, here's the path that worked for me:

1. **Choose single-ingredient foods:**
   - Eggs. Fish. Rice. Dairy. Steak. Fruit. Potatoes. Vegetables.
   - If it has a nutrition label, it's probably been engineered.
2. **Shop the perimeter of the grocery store:**
   - Produce section (fruits, vegetables), dairy section (eggs, yogurt, cheese), meat counter (real protein). Real food doesn't need fancy packaging.
3. **Read ingredients, not just the numbers on a label:**
   - If sugar is in the top three ingredients, it's dessert.
   - "Natural flavors" can mean over 50 chemicals.
   - More than five ingredients? Probably engineered.
4. **Reset your taste buds:**
   - Go 42 days without heavily processed food, starting with a couple of days at a time.

- Suddenly, real food tastes alive.

5. **Live by the 80/20 rule:**
    - 80% real, whole foods, 20% whatever you enjoy.

Perfection isn't the goal. Consistency and sustainability are.

The food industry spent decades learning how to keep us addicted. But in just 42 days, you can learn how to take back control. Most people try to fight back alone. Healthy people enjoy food without letting food control them.

That's the final key:

Be intentional with what goes in your body.

When you control what you eat, you take back more than your health. You take back

your life.

If you're ready to reclaim your energy, confidence, and health with a sustainable approach, I'd love to walk alongside you.

Ready to go from tired, embarrassed, and frustrated to energetic, admired, and vibrant health? Let's walk together.

Ready to join LIFE 42 Wellness?

Reach out. There is a second chance...and it begins now.

LIFE 42 Wellness
David Medansky
(602) 721-5218
davidmedansky@gmail.com

About The Author

FROM HEALTH CRISIS TO CLIMBING MOUNT KILIMANJARO

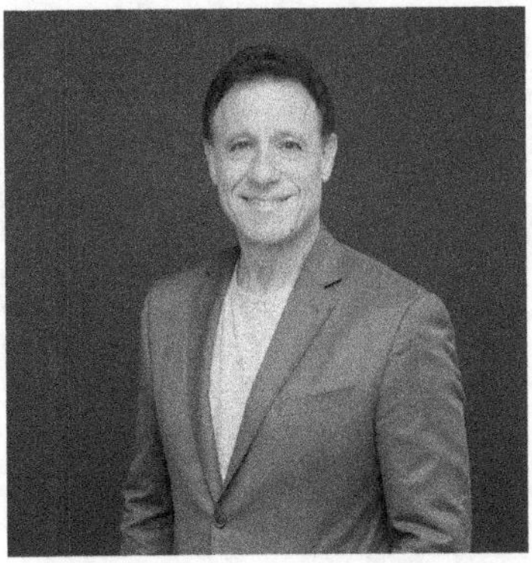

David Medansky, widely known as "The Health Guy," is a best-selling, multiple award-winning author, speaker, and founder of LIFE 42 Wellness.

After struggling with his own weight and health issues for years, David's life turned around when, at age 61, his doctor told him he had a 95% chance of a fatal heart attack unless he made immediate changes. In just four months, David shed 50 pounds, reversed his health risks, and has maintained a vibrant, healthy lifestyle ever since, without fad diets or extreme measures.

Drawing on an extensive background as a successful trial attorney and wellness advocate, David is dedicated to empowering others to regain energy, confidence, and wellbeing through simple, practical steps. He's inspired thousands through his books, workshops, and speaking engagements, including corporate and community events across the country.

At the age of 67, David accomplished the extraordinary feat of hiking to the summit of Mt. Kilimanjaro, proving it's never too late for a new beginning. His approachable, science-backed methods and relatable storytelling have helped countless people transform their lives—one healthy habit at a time.

David lives in Phoenix, sharing his journey and expertise with audiences everywhere.

To Book David Medansky for a Corporate Event,
Call (602) 721-5218

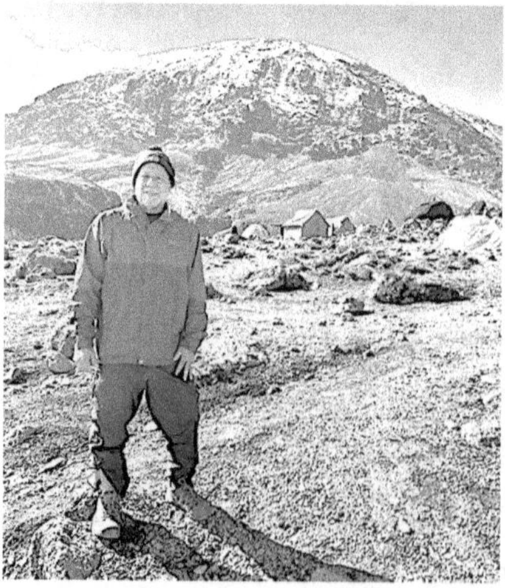

Other Books by David Medansky

If you enjoyed this book, you might also love:

Jaded Health

Break the Chains of Dieting

If Not Now, When?

Stop Dieting, Start Thinning

Discover Your Thinner Self

Coming Fall 2026: Echoes of Tomorrow

Coming Spring 2027: The Cost of $uccess

Coming Summer 2027: Seasoned

www.ingramcontent.com/pod-product-compliance
Lightning Source LLC
LaVergne TN
LVHW021036011026
849160LV00009BA/670